D1109512

THIRD EDITION

HYPNOSIS
for CHANGE

JOSIE HADLEY AND CAROL STAUDACHER

MJF BOOKS
NEW YORK

Publisher's Note: This publication is designed to provide accurate and authoritative information in regard to the subject matter covered. It is sold with the understanding that the publisher is not engaged in rendering psychological, financial, legal, or other professional services. If expert assistance or counseling is needed, the services of a competent professional should be sought.

Published by MJF Books
Fine Communications
Two Lincoln Square
60 West 66th Street
New York, NY 10023

Hypnosis for Change
Library of Congress Control No. 00-135233
ISBN 1-56731-392-2

This edition published by arrangement with New Harbinger Publications, Inc.

Text design by Tracy Marie Powell.

Manufactured in the United States of America on acid-free paper

MJF Books and the MJF colophon are trademarks of Fine Creative Media, Inc.

10   9   8   7   6   5   4   3   2   1

I would like to thank the wonderful people
I have met from coast to coast and abroad.
The support I have had and friendships
I have made through *Hypnosis for Change*
have truly been transformational. A special
thanks to Terry Attwood, Annette Krash Graff,
Simone, Lolly Piombi, and Dorthy V. Tyo,
who are truly my family of friends.

—*Josie Hadley*

To H.A.S., who can be depended upon to
read any manuscript as it evolves—any time,
anywhere. And for my daughter Susan,
whose smile mesmerizes.

—*Carol Staudacher*

With appreciation to Matthew McKay,
who should receive the Managing Editor
Laureate Award.

Contents

Introduction

In recent years, hypnosis has gained momentum and acceptance as part of the evolution of our health care system. The techniques of hypnosis are neither mysterious nor difficult. In this book, the "how to" is made completely accessible to everyone. All of the material presented here is designed to meet the needs of interested lay people, as well as professionals who use or would like to use hypnosis in their practice.

The first three chapters investigate the background of hypnosis, explore all the facets of the induction, and examine the various aspects of hypnotic communication. These chapters provide you with a solid foundation to understand the origins of hypnosis, its past and present uses, the techniques for its application, and the structure of any basic hypnotic induction. Also discussed are the qualities necessary for the hypnotic voice and the types of suggestions used in an hypnotic induction. Once these basic concepts are understood, you will be ready to use any of the eleven treatment chapters. If you are seeking treatment for yourself in a specific problem area—such as smoking, weight loss, stress, or lack of self-esteem—you can then turn to the specific treatment chapter which deals with that problem.

It is also possible that you may need to use a *combination* of treatment chapters in coping with some problems. For example, if you are a tennis player who is primarily interested in improving your game,

you will find help in Chapter 13, "Improving Your Athletic Performance." But if part of your problem on the court stems from a lack of
confidence or feelings of intimidation, you will also benefit from
Chapter 11, which deals with self-esteem. If you are working on ridding
yourself of a specific phobia, you may refer to Chapter 7, "Treating
Phobias." But since phobias can be caused or heightened by stress,
you will also benefit from the reinforcement offered in Chapter 6,
"Stress Reduction." Or perhaps you are anxious about an upcoming
surgical procedure. You can refer to the newly added Chapter 19,
"Surgery," as well as to Chapter 16, "Anxiety and Panic."

It is not realistic to think that *every* person's problem can be easily
solved by turning to a chapter having a title that corresponds to that
problem and using the information there without considering all the
aspects of the area you wish to improve. The treatment chapters do
serve as foundations for change, but don't rule out the treatment of
subsidiary problems that may be intensifying your major problem.

If you plan to use this book with your clients or patients, you
will follow the same approach. First, you will identify the major problem,
and then you will pinpoint other trouble areas that may be exacerbating
that problem.

The last two chapters in the book deal with topics most relevant
to people practicing hypnotherapy in a professional setting—to those
who are working with clients, patients, students, or employees. These
chapters discuss the practical aspects of the hypnotherapist/client relationship and cover situations likely to occur, as well as special techniques that may be used.

Hypnosis can be amazingly effective and often is directly responsible for major changes in an individual's life pattern. But it must be
stressed that it is not a guaranteed method of chasing away private
demons. Just as all people do not react in exactly the same way to
the same medical prescription, all people will not get identical results
from the same hypnotic induction. One person may respond very
quickly to the *Weight Loss Induction,* experiencing a gradual but noticeable weight loss. Another person may need to use the induction
over a period of seven months before a major weight reduction occurs.
One individual may get rid of a lifelong fear in a relatively short period
of time; another person with the same fear may need to work on stress
and self-esteem in addition to treating the fear itself, taking incremental
steps to achieve complete elimination of the phobia.

Of course, if you have physical symptoms or emotional problems
that are either prolonged or severe, consult a physician or therapist
and get an all-clear signal to go ahead with self-hypnosis. Obviously,
it would not be practical to use the chapter on health problems to
"cure" bleeding ulcers, or to employ the stress reduction chapter to
cope with an unwavering suicidal impulse.

These exceptions put aside, the use of this material will make it possible for you to establish a fresh outlook and a positive approach to problems, and it will provide you with the new skills necessary to alter old habits. In fact, by using the information in Chapters 2 and 3, you can create your own induction to treat any problem, no matter how unique.

One recent convert to hypnosis explained it this way: "Some days I am under tremendous pressure and must deal effectively with a lot of forces all at once. When these days occur, I use mini-inductions to drive away negative reactions and situations before they have a chance to magnify and become debilitating. I used to have frequent migraine headaches. I don't any more. I use hypnosis and don't allow a headache to happen."

As you first learn about and later explore self-hypnosis, you will determine the ways in which it can work best for you. Remember that every challenge offers a whole universe of new opportunities.

1

What Is Hypnosis?

Hypnosis has long been associated with the strange and mysterious, with sideshows and faith healers. But the truth is that hypnosis isn't the least bit mysterious or supernatural. In fact, you have been in an hypnotic state literally thousands of times. You didn't notice it because it seemed such a natural state of mind. And the hypnotic state *is* natural for all humans and many animals.

Chances are, at one time or another, you have found yourself driving along a familiar freeway *past* your exit, or perhaps you suddenly became aware of yourself behind the wheel and wondered where you were going. Occurrences such as these are common. Let's take a look at what makes them possible.

Everything you have learned is stored in your subconscious. Because you have already learned to drive, your driving skill is stored in your subconscious. As you begin your journey, you get in your car, maneuver out onto the freeway, move into a continuous flow of traffic, and reach a consistent speed. Now your conscious mind is free. That is, because the knowledge required for driving exists in your subconscious, your conscious mind drifts off, allowing your subconscious to become more active. You may become so engrossed in your thoughts that you drive in the direction of your office when your actual destination is the grocery store or the movie theater. When your attention is needed to change lanes, avoid something in the road, stop at a toll gate, or slow for an offramp, your conscious mind comes into play again. You may even arrive at your destination and wonder how you got there so quickly.

Driving is only one automatic activity. Whenever you do anything automatic, your conscious mind is diverted from your subconscious and you are more likely to go into an hypnotic state, such as the one described. Some of your automatic activities are more apt than others to allow or provide daydreaming. For example, your mind might drift when you are dining alone, taking a shower, mowing your lawn, or jogging. These activities, like driving, are stored in your subconscious. While you are functioning in this automatic mode, it is quite easy to drift from an alert state into a different level of consciousness. Daydreaming is the first of the levels in a trance state.

Levels of Consciousness

The levels of consciousness range from a state of alertness to a sleep state. *There are no rigid boundaries setting off one level from the next.* Instead, the levels blend into each other and can be generally defined, as shown in the following chart.

LEVEL OF CONSCIOUSNESS	MENTAL AND PHYSICAL CHARACTERISTICS	EXAMPLE OF ACTIVITY
Alert	1. Normal intellectual functioning. 2. Normal reflexive and and motor response.	You are playing tennis.
Daydreaming: Light Trance	1. Relaxation of body. 2. Slowed breathing and pulse. 3. Withdrawal into self. 4. Direction of attention to imagined activity, dialogue, or event which may be possible or impossible.	You are idly thinking about playing a game of tennis.
Moderate Trance	1. Loss of awareness of surroundings. 2. Closed eyes. 3. Increased awareness of internal functions, such as heartbeat or breathing. 4. Increased receptivity of senses. 5. Intensified imagery. 6. Literal interpretation of speech. (If asked, "Would you lift your arm?" you would answer, "Yes.")	You are imagining yourself on tennis court playing a game.

Deep Trance	1. Further reduction of activity and energy output.	You physically feel yourself playing tennis.
	2. Limpness or stiffness of limbs.	
	3. Narrowing of attention.	
	4. Increased suggestibility.	
	5. Illusions of senses possible.	
	6. Loss of auditory receptivity and environmental awareness.	
	7. Heightened function of creative process.	
Sleep	1. Suspension of voluntary exercise.	You dream of participating in a tennis match.
	2. Severe reduction or absence of conscious thought.	

The three middle levels are the ones in which behavior modification will occur and the ones in which you will be most susceptible to posthypnotic suggestion. But it is important to understand that no two individuals will have identical experiences as they progress from the state of alertness to the deep trance. You may be far more suggestible in a moderate trance than your friend is in a deep trance. It is even possible for someone in a light trance to accept a major suggestion, such as numbness in a body part.

But generally speaking, when you are in a trance state in which you are receptive to hypnotic suggestion, you will be likely to experience relaxation, sleepiness, a rigidity or limpness in the muscles of your arms and legs, skin warmth or coldness, sensations of tingling or feelings of electricity, and narrowness of attention.

It is also common to have a sense of strangeness or unreality. This means that you may see yourself or your surroundings in a new way, more detached or more connected than usual. One subject described his feelings this way: "I felt as if my mind were floating above my physical body." A second described her trance by saying, "My entire body felt as if it were made of warm, bendable plastic that I could mold and shape." Another said, "The windows of the room seemed to squint shut like eyes, and then I was in a very comfortable, pleasant darkness." Some subjects will not have any sensations similar to these. The way each person responds depends upon his attitudes, preconceived ideas, expectations, and sometimes fantasies.

As you examine the various mental and physical characteristics of the trance states shown on the chart, you will see why hypnosis has been associated, in varying degrees, with mystery and awe.

From Shamans to Sigmund: Origins of Hypnosis

Every culture has used hypnosis in one form or another. The earliest evidence of its existence was found among shamans, who were also referred to as "witch doctors," "medicine men," or "healers."

In preparation for healing, a shaman adhered to certain practices that allowed his powers of concentration to be heightened. He avoided the use of chemical or alcoholic substances for 24 hours prior to the healing session. Because the shaman needed to feel strongly focused, he placed himself in an environment that was not distracting in any way—a dark, quiet room, an isolated place in the forest, or a cave. There, the shaman made himself as comfortable as possible and began his descent into the "lower world." This often meant visualizing an opening in the earth and a journey downward into that opening. The journey was frequently helped by the accompaniment of drum beats, chanting, singing, or dancing, aids that could be provided by the shaman's companion or by the shaman himself. The accompanying activities all had two qualities in common: They were rhythmic and monotonous. The repetition and constancy allowed the shaman's subconscious mind to become strongly focused, seek out the sick spirit of the patient, make it whole, and bring it back to him. The shaman actually engaged in a powerful process of visualization and suggestion during which he willed the sick person to be healed.

In the 1700s, an Austrian doctor, Franz Anton Mesmer (1733-1815), recognized this ancient healing phenomenon and incorporated it into a theory of animal magnetism. Mesmer believed that a "cosmic fluid" could be stored in inanimate objects, such as magnets, and transferred to patients to cure them of illness.

Mesmer dressed flamboyantly. His consulting rooms were dimly lighted and hung with mirrors. Soft music broke the otherwise deep silence. The doctor's patients sat in a circle around a vat, which contained such elements as powdered glass or iron filings. The patients held onto iron rods that came out of the vat and were supposed to transmit the curing force.

Mesmer's first big success was with a 29-year-old woman who suffered from a convulsive malady, a condition commonly labeled a "nervous disorder." Her symptoms consisted of blood rushing to her head and a tremendous pain in her ears and head. This state was followed by delirium, rage, vomiting, and fainting.

During one of the young woman's attacks, Mesmer applied three magnets to the patient's stomach and legs while she quieted and concentrated on the positive effects of the "cosmic fluid." In just a short time, her symptoms subsided. When her symptoms surfaced again the next day, Mesmer gave her another treatment and achieved similar results.

Mesmer believed that the "cosmic fluid," stimulated by the magnets, was directed through his patient's body. Her energy flow was restored, and as a result she regained her health.

Eventually Mesmer discarded the magnets. He began to regard himself as a magnet through which a fluid life force could be conducted and then transmitted to others as a healing force. This is what Mesmer called "animal magnetism."

Despite the fact that no evidence supports the existence of Mesmer's "cosmic fluids" and "animal magnetism," he had a tremendous rate of success. Thousands of sick but hopeful people flocked to his treatment center. The only explanation for his successes is that his patients were literally "mesmerized" into the belief and expectation that they would be cured. *Mesmerism* became the forerunner of hypnotic suggestion.

During this same period a new twist on Mesmer's theories was introduced by one of his disciples, the marquis de Puysegur. He believed that the "cosmic fluid" was not magnetic, but electric. This electric fluid was generated in all living things — in plants as well as animals. Puysegur used the natural environment to fill his patients with the healing electric fluid that was expected to end their suffering. His clinic was held outdoors, where the sick were received under an elm tree in the center of the village green. Puysegur believed that the tree had an innate healing power and that the force would travel through the trunk and branches to cords that he hung from the tree. At the foot of the tree, patients sat in a circle on stone benches with the cords wrapped around the diseased parts of their bodies. They were "connected" to each other by touching their thumbs together, which made it possible for the "fluid" to circulate from person to person and to heal.

During this activity, Puysegur noticed a strange phenomenon. Some of the patients entered a somnambulistic state (a deep sleep) as a result of being mesmerized. In this state, the patient could still communicate and be lucid and responsive to the suggestions of the mesmerist. The marquis had discovered the hypnotic trance, but had not identified it as such.

In the mid 1800s, the hypnotic trance was used to relieve pain. A leading London physician, John Elliotson (1791–1868), reported 1,834 surgical operations performed painlessly. In India, a Scottish surgeon named James Esdaile (1808–1859) performed many major operations, such as the amputation of limbs, using mesmerism (or, as he called it, a "magnetic sleep") as the sole anesthetic. One procedure involved conditioning the patient weeks before the surgery was to occur. This was accomplished by inducing a trance state in the patient and offering posthypnotic suggestions to numb the part of the body on which the surgery was to be performed. In a second method, the hypnotist attended to the patient in the operating room, inducing a trance state and suggesting disassociation from any pain. It was possible for the patient to be completely lucid during this state and also be oblivious to pain, as if he had been completely anesthetized.

Mesmerism continued to provoke new theories and uses. During the late 1800s, an English physician, James Braid (1795–1860), gave mesmerism a scientific explanation. He believed mesmerism to be a "nervous sleep" and coined the word *hypnosis,* derived from the Greek word *hypnos,* meaning sleep. Braid showed that hypnotized subjects are often abnormally susceptible to impressions on the senses and that much of the subjects' behavior was due to suggestions made verbally.

Soon other theories began to emerge. Jean Martin Charcot (1825–1893), a neurologist who taught in Paris, explained hypnosis as a state of hysteria and categorized it as an abnormal neurological activity.

In France, Auguste Ambroise Leibeault (1823–1904) and Hippolyte Bernheim (1837–1919) were the first to regard hypnosis as a *normal* phenomenon. They asserted that expectation is a most important factor in the induction of hypnosis, that increased suggestibility is its essential symptom, and that the hypnotist works on the patient by mental influences.

As hypnosis began to receive serious study and could be explained rationally, it began to gain acceptance. It was no longer relegated to the bizarre.

Freud became interested in hypnosis at this same time and visited Leibeault and Bernheim's clinic to learn their induction techniques. As Freud observed patients enter an hypnotic state, he began to recognize the existence of the unconscious. Although he was not the first to make this observation, he was the first to recognize the unconscious as a major source of psychopathology. Early in his research, however, Freud rejected hypnosis as the tool to unlock repressed memories, favoring instead his techniques of free association and dream interpretation. With the rise of psychoanalysis in the first half of this century, hypnosis declined in popularity.

But a reversal occurred. Beginning in the 1950s, hypnosis experienced a rebirth as researchers found new and potent uses for it in therapy. The trance state is now being recognized as a highly effective tool for modifying behavior and for healing.

Making Hypnosis Work for You

What can hypnosis do for you, other than provide a fascinating new experience? What can you gain from it?

The answer is that hypnosis can be used to improve your general functioning — to make you feel better mentally or physically.

You may also be concerned about what hypnosis can do *to* you.

Hypnosis is not in any way harmful, but it is completely understandable for a beginning hypnotic subject to have some reservations. You may want to ask a few questions to assuage your curiosity and allay your fears. The questions which follow are representative of those most frequently asked of hypnotherapists:

> When I am in a trance can you make me cluck like a chicken? Bark like a dog? Act like a newborn baby?

> Will I tell you something I've never told anyone? Will I talk about things that are private?

> Could I stay "frozen" in one position and never come out of it?

> Could I harm myself?

What these questions are getting at is this: Can a hypnotist make you do something that is embarrassing, shocking, or irreversible? No, you will not do anything you do not think is acceptable. That is, you cannot be "made" to violate your own values or accepted patterns of behavior.

It is important for you to remember that a trance state can be terminated by you at any time. It is your choice to enter the trance state, and you can always choose to leave it. If you were left in a trance state by your hypnotherapist or by your hypnotic tape, you would either return to full consciousness on your own or enter a natural sleep and awaken after a pleasant nap. No one has ever disappeared for long.

Now that you know the trance state is safe territory, you can examine the ways in which it can be used. Listed below are some of the basic beneficial functions most commonly associated with hypnotherapy. Of course, individuals' needs vary. Because of this, there are as many applications as there are hypnotic subjects. Included here are only a few of the specific applications that hypnotherapists regularly employ.

BENEFICIAL FUNCTION	APPLICATION OF FUNCTION
Produces anesthesia in the body.	A patient visiting the dentist can anesthetize his own mouth, cheek, and gums to greatly reduce or eliminate pain.
Improves sleep, reduces stress, controls painful symptoms.	A chronic insomniac can reduce or eliminate stress and reprogram his subconscious to improve the quality and duration of his sleep.
Controls some organic functions such as bleeding and heart rate.	A person who suffers from high blood pressure can slow his own pulse rate and reduce his own blood pressure.

Makes possible partial age regression: reliving an experience in the distant past, just as it occurred, with the senses operating as they did at the time of the original experience.	A person may eliminate an irrational fear of something such as spiders, dogs, enclosed space, or bridges; may reduce fear of intimate relationships which resulted from the trauma of incest during childhood.
Develops abnormal abilities of concentration: increases capacity to learn and remember in enormous detail.	A student can prepare for an examination by assimilating and retaining a vast amount of material that can be recalled at will.
Compresses a great deal of thinking and recall into a very short amount of real time.	A subject can review the events of his life, find a scene, and set the stage for a particular situation that needs change.

As you can see, all of the functions listed have to do with your own thinking and actions. In all of the applications — whether it be numbing your gums or driving over a bridge — you are the controlling factor. It is always through your own effort that change occurs. This change can affect your life minimally, or it can make a dramatic difference in your lifestyle, success, and feeling of well-being.

Because you know in which areas of your life you need direction, assistance, or motivation, you can assess your personal needs and select a corresponding self-hypnosis treatment. Following is a summary of the specialized hypnosis treatments presented in this manual.

Weight loss. Motivates weight loss, reprograms eating habits, and establishes a procedure for weight maintenance.

Smoking. Eliminates the smoking habit and provides procedures for permanent behavior modification.

Stress. Employs techniques to reduce or eliminate stress, promotes relaxation, and reprograms specific behavior patterns.

Phobias. Eliminates a fear of something, such as riding in an elevator, air travel, crowds, or disease.

Natural childbirth. Supports and reinforces Bradley and Lamaze methods, programs pain control, establishes communication with the child, and promotes a positive postbirth phase.

Major health problems. Eases the symptoms and reduces the effects of such chronic problems as colitis, muscle spasms, and ulcers.

Pain. Controls pain in chronic conditions such as arthritis or back pain; introduces techniques for reducing pain of surgery, injury, or disease.

Self-esteem and motivation. Improves self-projection, reprograms past negative behavior, increases confidence and self-acceptance; programs for specific goals, instills feelings of comfort in regard to success.

Learning. Improves study habits, enhances memory, instills positive attitude toward learning, and incorporates reward.

Sports. Refines athletic performance by allowing strong focus on areas that need improvement, creates a sense of success in the execution of skills, increases stamina and coordination, puts the competitive spirit in perspective, and enhances overall attitude.

Creativity. Releases blocked potential in areas of writing, painting, and the performing arts; motivates production and promotes the use of the trance state as an aid to insight.

Sleep. Breaks bad nighttime habits, restructures pre-bedtime mental activity.

Anxiety and panic. Teaches how to relax in the middle of a panic attack, stop thoughts that produce panic attacks, replace thoughts with positive coping statements, accept all feelings and sensations.

Child abuse. Releases negative patterns, increases feelings of self-worth, heals the inner child.

Loss and separation. Addresses physical symptoms of the separation reaction, removes blocks to recovery, releases pent-up emotions, heals emotional wounds.

Surgery. Eases anxiety about surgery, explores the possibility of surgical procedures without chemical anesthesia.

Depression. Overrides the negative thoughts that contribute to depression, leads the way to a more positive outlook.

In addition to these areas, you will also learn how to design an induction that meets other exclusive or unique needs. No matter how special your problem is, it can be successfully reduced or eliminated by the thoughtful application of hypnosis.

2

The Hypnotic Induction

At this point, you probably find yourself in one of these two states of mind: (1) You want to participate in hypnosis, but have some reservations about *how* or *if* it will work for you. Or (2) You acknowledge your need for hypnotic treatment and are ready, perhaps even eager, to improve some specific area of your life. In either case, you are a potential hypnotic subject. As such, you are no doubt curious about how the individual you are *at this very moment* can be transported into the realm where hypnotic suggestion is possible.

Measuring Your Suggestibility

To get an indication of your response level, you may measure your own suggestibility by using one of the three exercises below. You may guide yourself through the exercise, or have someone say it to you.

STIFF ARM EXERCISE

Make sure you are completely comfortable. Stretch your legs, your arms. And now begin to relax. Close your eyes and take a deep breath . . . and exhale . . . and relax. Completely relax. Relax your legs, lower back, relax your shoulders. Relax your shoulders, your arms, your neck, your face. Relax your whole body, just relax. Take another deep breath . . . and exhale . . . let go, and relax. Become aware of the rhythm of your breathing. Begin to flow with the rhythm of your breathing, and as you inhale, relax your breathing and begin to feel your body drift and float into relaxation. The sounds around you are unimportant, let them go, and relax. Let every muscle in your body completely relax from the top of your head to the tips of your toes. As you inhale gently, relax. As you exhale, release any tension, any stress from any part of your body, mind and thoughts.

Now raise one arm in front of you. Hold it out straight. Close your fist and make it very tight, your fist tight, and now your arm is getting stiff, it's getting stiffer, it's getting very, very stiff. Your arm is stiff, very, very stiff. Your whole arm is stiff from your shoulder to your fist. Your arm is straight and hard and will not bend. You try to bend your arm, and it becomes more stiff. Your stiff arm is still and straight and nothing moves it. Nothing can move it, it is completely stiff from your shoulder to your fist, completely stiff. Your arm is completely stiff. Now I will count from five to one. When I say five you will begin to relax your arm. As you hear each number you will relax your arm more and more, then when I say one your arm will be completely relaxed at your side. Five . . . begin to relax your arm . . . four . . . feel your arm relax . . . three . . . relax . . . two . . . one. Your arm is completely relaxed.

The degree to which you respond freely and easily indicates your suggestibility. If your arm became stiff and remained stiff until the count of five began, you are a suggestible subject.

THE BUCKET EXERCISE

[Repeat the first paragraph of the Stiff Arm Exercise to achieve relaxation.]

Stretch your arms in front of you at a level even with your shoulders. Imagine you are holding a bucket in each hand. Curl your fingers around the handles of the buckets, hold onto those two buckets. The bucket in your left hand is made of paper, it is made of paper. It is empty and feels very light, the bucket in your left hand feels very, very light. The bucket in your left hand is very, very light because it is made of paper. You hold that light bucket in your left hand. The bucket in your right hand is made of iron. It is made of iron, it is made of heavy, heavy iron, and the bucket has a few rocks in it. As you hold the heavy iron bucket, more and more rocks are dropped into the bucket until the bucket is completely full of heavy rocks. The bucket is completely full of heavy rocks, the rocks are heaped up to the top of the bucket. The bucket is so very heavy, it is pulling your right arm down. The bucket of rocks pulls your arm down and your arm goes down because the heavy iron bucket is so heavy, so very heavy.

In this exercise, your arms will have begun to move some distance from their original position at shoulder level. The further the distance between the left and right arm, the greater your suggestibility.

THE HAND CLASP EXERCISE
[Repeat the first paragraph of the Stiff Arm Exercise to achieve relaxation.]

Clasp your hands in front of you and push them tightly together. Push them together very tightly. As you hold them tightly, imagine that a very strong, strong glue has been spread on your hands and the glue is beginning to dry, hard and fast. It is drying and keeping your hands together, your hands are tight together. Your hands no longer feel as if they are two separate hands. They are one. Your fingers and palms are glued together, hard and fast, very hard and fast. You test to see how strongly the glue is holding your hands, and you find your hands, the palms of your hands, your fingers are stuck together. They are stuck together. They are glued together so tightly they feel as one. They are glued together very, very tightly and feel as one. On the count of three you will be unable to pull your hands apart. The harder you try to pull them apart, the more they will stick together. They will stick together more each time you hear a number. One . . . two . . . three.

These exercises measured your receptivity and responsiveness to suggestion. The greater your suggestibility, the more receptive a hypnotic candidate you will be. An extreme response does not guarantee that you will accept and act on the hypnotic suggestions you are given for modifying your behaviour, but it does mean that you will be a good receptor—and being a good receptor is the first step toward successful hypnotic treatment.

Induction Styles

The real vehicle for change is the induction, which produces, or causes, an hypnotic state. You may think of the induction as an ocean liner that is going to carry you from the mainland to an island. The mainland is your conscious mind, the island your subconscious. It is on that island that you will experience peacefulness and relaxation. There you will also be given the "code" you need to break your current behavior pattern and replace it with one that is more desirable.

There are several kinds of inductions, varying in approach, length of time, and tone. They can be commanding or permissive. This chapter will explore different syles of induction and the ways they work. It is important to understand, however, that although inductions may be quite different from one another, they must all bring about these results:

- Relaxation of body and mind
- Narrowed focus of attention
- Reduced awareness of external environment and everyday concerns
- Greater internal awareness of sensations
- A trance state

The Fixation Induction draws attention to a very narrow point of interest such as a swinging watch or pendulum, a dot on the wall, or a candle. As concentration focuses on the fixation point, your attention is drawn away from external sights and sounds and directly to the object. This induction may take seconds, or it may take twenty or thirty minutes, depending on your suggestibility.

To use this induction, you get in a comfortable position, light a candle, and stare into the flame as it burns and flickers. Your complete attention should be given to the flame. The induction begins like this:

Watch the flame burn and flicker and keep your eyes on the flame and concentrate on it. Watch the flame flicker and keep your eyes on the flame. As you watch the flame burning, your eyes will become heavy, become heavy, and your eyes will grow heavier and heavier . . . and heavier . . . heavier . . . until they close.

The Rapid Induction produces a trance state very quickly. This induction consists of short, rapid commands, such as the following:

Close your eyes. Lower your head until your chin meets your chest. Raise your arm to shoulder level. When your arm feels very light and floats, you will then be in a trance.

This induction is most successful with highly suggestible subjects. Others may find it too abrupt and not relaxing.

The *Rapid Induction* is most closely associated with the theatricality of hypnosis. That is, a hypnotist who is giving a demonstration can give a suggestibility test to an audience to quickly determine the suggestibility of individual members of the audience. He can then use the *Rapid Induction* with these highly responsive subjects to produce a dramatic demonstration.

A therapist in private practice may, after working with a subject a few times, determine that the person is highly suggestible. The therapist might then use the *Rapid Induction* as a time-saver when working with that particular subject.

The Indirect Induction differs from all others in that it does not use any directives. Instead, the induction communicates through the use of analogies or metaphors. This approach to hypnosis works particularly well with subjects who would resist other more direct approaches. The reason for this is simple: It is difficult for the subject to resist or reject a suggestion that he does not know he is receiving.

As an example, in an *Indirect Induction* an analogy could be drawn between the *heart* and a *water pump*. If a hypnotherapist were dealing with a subject who was undergoing hypnotic treatment for an irregular heartbeat due to stress, the therapist could then talk about how the old-fashioned water pump was manipulated by the strong old farmer who used it, how the pump was dependable and worked better when the farmer pumped water at a regular, rhythmic pace.

If a therapist were working with a child who had a sleepwalking problem, he might tell a story about a hibernating bear, discussing the bear's need for warmth and sleep and the comfort the animal derived from the long rest.

For an older child who was having trouble fitting into a group, who could not participate in group activities and was continually disruptive, the hypnotherapist might describe the way migrating birds often fly in formation, how they move together, how each bird in the flock seems to take up an equal amount of space. He might focus on the way each bird maintains the same rhythm and speed, allowing the flock to move as one whole, harmoniously and beautifully.

Milton Erickson, a master in the field of metaphor, worked successfully with patients exhibiting a wide range of symptoms. In one case, he dealt with a patient who was leading a metaphoric life. The young man draped himself in a sheet and went about the hospital ward claiming to be Jesus. Erickson approached the man and said, "I understand you have had experience as a carpenter?" When the patient replied that he had, Erickson gave him a project to complete. He instructed him to build a bookcase. In this way, the patient, working within his own metaphor, was shifted into productive labor, one of the major steps in his recovery.

The Relaxation Induction systematically relaxes every muscle in your body. The relaxation may begin at the top of the head and work down, or it may begin with the toes and work upwards. The induction is simple and easy to use when hypnotizing others or doing self-hypnosis. It begins this way:

> *Take a nice deep breath, close your eyes and begin to relax. Just think about relaxing every muscle in your body, from the top of your head to the tip of your toes.*

Since this is the basic induction and the one that is the most widely used, it will be explored in detail later in this chapter.

The Progressive Relaxation Induction is designed to meet the needs of those who find it difficult to relax. It is used extensively in the area of stress management and incorporates both physical and mental relaxation. It takes an estimated 30 to 40 minutes, compared to between 20 and 25 minutes for the classic *Relaxation Induction,* mentioned briefly above.

This induction is popular with people who need to relax specific areas of the body to relieve chronic tension in shoulders, chest, legs, or elsewhere. The *Progressive Relaxation Induction* relaxes the major muscles of the body one at a time, concentrating first on a tense neck, then shoulders, then lower back, and so on. When using it, you can start at your head and progress down your body, or begin at your feet, or at any other body area. You may want to begin at the particular spot in your body where you feel the most tension so that tension can be eliminated before progressing to other areas. It would be difficult for you to experience relaxation in the shoulders, for example, if you had a knotted muscle in your upper arm. A *Progressive Relaxation Induction* could begin like this:

> *Make yourself comfortable. Concentrate on your right shoulder and tense your right shoulder.* [PAUSE.] *Now relax your right shoulder.* [PAUSE AND REPEAT THREE TIMES.] *Now concentrate on your left shoulder. Tighten your left shoulder.* [PAUSE.] *Now relax your left shoulder.* [PAUSE AND REPEAT THREE TIMES.] *Now concentrate on your right arm. . .*

Regardless of where you begin, each major muscle in each body area is tightened and relaxed three times. By the time the whole body has been covered, you should be completely relaxed.

Hypnotic Techniques

Two main techniques are used for the induction process: the *authoritarian technique* and the *permissive technique.* The characteristics of each differ drastically, and each one tends to be more effective in different situations and with different subjects.

The authoritarian technique is commanding and direct. Its purpose is to establish control over the subject and alter behavior through the use of repetitious commands.

This approach was used in early experiments because hypnotists believed that the authority they had over their subjects increased their chance for success. To some degree, this still holds true today. If the subject views the hypnotist as an authority figure, the subject may have greater confidence in the power of an induction. The heightened expectation alone increases the chances for success. Here is an example of an authoritarian technique:

> [SPEAK FIRMLY.] *You will listen to my voice and my voice will help you to relax very deeply. I want you to relax deeply. As you relax deeper and deeper you will respond to the suggestion I give you.* You will now stop smoking. You will now stop smoking. *This is your wish and your desire and you will act on it* now.

Generally speaking, the subjects who are most responsive to the authoritarian technique are those who have great respect for and respond well to authoritarian figures in daily life, such as teachers, parents, employers, community leaders, and police officers. People who are scientifically oriented will be more likely to fit into this category, as opposed to those who are highly imaginative or creative.

This technique works best in individual sessions and is difficult to use in a group situation.

The symptoms that may be treated using this technique are often related to a repressed emotion (for example, obesity which started at a young age because of the birth of a brother or sister and the resulting need to gain parental attention). Since the problem originated in a childhood response to authority, the authoritarian technique is employed to take the subject back in time so that he or she can see the problem, understand it, and let go of the need for the behavior that compensates for it. An authoritarian figure played a major role in the *cause* of the problem; therefore, another authoritarian figure can help *unlock* the problem, and eventually eliminate it.

Any fear that began during childhood, such as fear of being alone or fear of the dark, can be reduced or eliminated by regressing through the authoritarian technique.

This technique also works well with a subject who is responding to a mate as if he or she were a parent. As this technique is used, a suggestion is given to the subject to assume responsibility and eliminate dependent behavior. This is done during the induction by increasing the self-confidence of the subject and reprogramming independent behavior.

The permissive technique employs a softer tone of voice to lull the subject into relaxation. In contrast to the authoritarian technique, the hypnotist and the subject are equal partners in the process. More imagery is used to enhance suggestions, and greater responsibility is given to the subject. Here is an example of this technique:

> [SOFTLY SPOKEN.] *As you listen to my voice let it help you to relax. As you relax deeper and deeper, just imagine yourself in a peaceful place. It may be by the ocean or in the mountains. Any place is fine. Imagine how great you feel in the place. Now let*

yourself relax deeper, and as you relax deeper your desire to feel healthy and free of any habit grows strong, then stronger, and soon you realize you truly are a nonsmoker.

The subjects who are most responsive to this technique are ones who are more imaginative and creative. Because more specific, individualized imagery is incorporated into the induction, the induction becomes more real, more applicable to the individual.

This technique is particularly successful with subjects who are reaching goals, such as those people who want to become more successful in an occupation or who want to improve their working conditions through their own behavior.

The Language of an Induction

The language of an induction is designed to communicate opinions, thoughts, and feelings. It focuses your attention on yourself, your inner experiences, and your body. It helps you to become absorbed into the realm of imagination and to communicate below the level of consciousness. The following are key components of the language of induction.

Synonyms. Instead of using only one descriptive word exclusively, synonyms are used for reinforcement when describing the desired state. They strengthen the suggestions. For example, "You are feeling at ease, relaxed, calm, comfortable."

Paraphrased suggestions. Suggestions are repeated and paraphrased to enhance comprehension and ensure retention. For example, "Feel the relaxation flow through your body, feel the warmth of relaxation, relaxing every muscle in your body, feel all the muscles in your body relax."

Connective words. Connective words have two functions: (1) to maintain a steady flow so the monologue will not be interrupted, and (2) to precede a directive, such as "*and* now relax, feel all the muscles relax now *and* breathe deeply now *and* just relax all the muscles in your arms *and* because you are relaxed feel a warmth flow through your body . . . " In this context, the connective word *and* is a cue to respond.

Time designations. Words that specify time are used for stress and emphasis. They can signal the time the suggestion begins or the time it ends. For example, any of the following cues could be used to signal the beginning of a suggestion: "And *now at this very moment* release all tension from your body." "*In just a few moments* you will experience total relaxation." "*In the morning* you will awaken refreshed and relaxed." The end of a suggestion might be signaled by *"At the end of two hours* you will *stop* studying and this will end your test preparation."

The Hypnotic Voice

At one time or another, you have probably had the experience of being bored or lulled by a public speaker. No matter how hard you tried, it was impossible to concentrate. You repeatedly brought yourself back to the situation and forced yourself to listen carefully to each word; yet, quite against your will, your mind drifted. It drifted because the speaker's voice was putting you into a trance state. There are, in fact, certain people whose voices have a tone, volume, and lack of inflection that make them highly hypnotic.

Because the voice alone can elicit a trance state, the voice you use for your induction is extremely important to your entire hypnotic experience. The voice can be forceful and commanding, or it can be soothing and melodic. Before you record your own induction, consider the following characteristics of the hypnotic voice.

The voice for the basic induction is usually one of two types: *monotone* or *rhythmic.*

The *monotone voice* allows your attention to become inwardly focused because there is nothing distracting or diverting. The monotone is without inflection or variety in pitch or volume. It drones, "You will continue to relax, and now let all of the muscles in your forehead relax, and feel those muscles smooth, smooth and relaxed, and rest your eyes."

The *rhythmic* or *singsong voice* rocks you to peacefulness and lulls you into a trance. With this voice, the stresses in the sentences can be anticipated. They set up a rhythmic pattern that is comforting, soothing and predictable. For example, " . . . *dee*per, *dee*per, *dee*per into *to*tal relax*a*tion . . . " or *"Now* you are relax*ing all the *mus*cles in your *back.*"

There are other elements within the basic delivery that are important. They are used infrequently throughout the induction and can be interspersed with the basic voice, which is either *monotone* or *rhythmic.* These elements are as follows:

Word distortion for emphasis and reinforcement. Words are sometimes distorted to achieve a special, desired effect. For example, "Feel those muscles *loooose* and relaxed, feel those calf muscles *loooose* and relaxed, they are so *loooose* they feel like rubber bands." This type of word distortion is particularly beneficial to use during a Progressive Relaxation Induction if you have a particularly hard time relaxing and getting comfortable.

Raised pitch. The whole level of the voice changes with raised pitch. This elevated pitch, which penetrates the relaxed state of mind that has been produced by the monotone or rhythmic voice, is used to give a suggestion. The pitch allows an emphasis to be placed on posthypnotic suggestions such as "and *now you will stop smoking!*" It is also used to give a command to come up from an induction, such as "seven, eight, nine, ten, and *open your eyes* and come *all the way back, feeling great!*"

Uninterrupted rhythm. The uninterrupted rhythm is established through the use of connective words. You are pulled along the induction path by one continuous thread of speech. For example, "Feel yourself relax and continue to relax and just relax deeper and feel your entire body relaxing deeper and deeper . . . " This continuous flow of words establishes a rhythm that pulls you into the trance and closes out any distractions. It does not allow any opportunity for your attention to be diverted.

Silent pause. To allow time for you to respond to a suggestion or command, the silent pause is used. For example, "Now take a deep breath. [*Pause.*] Now exhale. [*Pause.*]" The pause is also used throughout the Progressive Relaxation Induction. "Concentrate on your right foot and tighten your right foot. [*Pause.*] Now relax your right foot. [*Pause.*]" It is absolutely necessary to allow adequate time for each response. Without it, you will feel anxious or hurried, and total relaxation will be impossible.

The Anatomy of an Induction

The best way to understand the art of hypnosis is to dissect an induction, analyze the wording and phrasing, and identify the desired results.

STEP 1. BEGINNING THE INDUCTION
Take a nice deep breath, close your eyes, and begin to relax. Just think about relaxing every muscle in your body . . .

As you begin to focus attention on your breathing and inner sensations, your awareness of external surroundings will decrease. By breathing deeply, you become aware of your internal sensations. You introduce your body to relaxation. The results are that your pulse slows, your breathing slows, you begin to withdraw, and you can direct your attention to the suggestions that are given to you.

STEP 2. SYSTEMATIC RELAXATION OF THE BODY
And begin by letting all the muscles in your face relax, especially your jaw; let your teeth part just a little bit and relax this area . . .

As you concentrate on relaxing every muscle in your body, your mind will also become more relaxed. You will experience an increased awareness of internal functions and an increased receptivity of the senses.

STEP 3. CREATING IMAGERY OF DEEPER RELAXATION
Drift and float into a deeper and deeper level of total relaxation. Feel a heavy, heavy weight being lifted off your shoulders...

The image of drifting down deeper and deeper helps you to enter a deeper trance. The tension in your shoulders is released as the "weight" is lifted from your shoulders. Any difference in your bodily sensations will support the suggestion that a change is taking place.

To create a feeling of lightness, the following image could be used.

You are feeling lighter and lighter, floating up higher and higher into a comfortable state of relaxation.

The direction, upward or downward, that is specified in the induction does not matter as long as it makes it possible for you to experience a change in your physical feelings.

STEP 4. DEEPENING THE TRANCE
Imagine a beautiful staircase. There are ten steps, and the ten steps lead you to a special and peaceful and beautiful place. In a moment I'm going to count backwards from ten to one, and you can imagine taking the steps down, and as you take each step feel your body relax more and more, feel it just drift down, down each step, and relax even deeper, ten, relax even deeper, nine... eight... seven... six... five... four... three... two ... one... deeper, deeper...

In order to further deepen your trance state, a count is used that usually goes from ten to one. You count *backwards* from ten to one as your trance deepens and *forward* from one to ten as you return to full consciousness. (These two major stages of the induction are referred to later in this chapter as *Going Down* and *Coming Up*.)

Although the image of a staircase was used above, you can substitute any image you like in order to enhance the feeling of going down. You may want to use the image of an elevator descending ten floors, as follows:

You are in an elevator and feel yourself begin to descend. As you watch the numbers of the floors passing, you see the number ten... and now the number nine...

At this stage a limpness or stiffness of your limbs will occur. Your attention will have narrowed, and your suggestibility will heighten. You will also experience an intensification of the creative process. The surrounding environment will be closed out.

STEP 5. THE SPECIAL PLACE
And now imagine a peaceful and special place. You can imagine this special place or perhaps you can even feel it. You are in a . . . [INSERT A DESCRIPTION OF YOUR SPECIAL PLACE.] You are alone and there is no one to disturb you. This is the most peaceful place in the world for you.

The special place you choose will be one that is unique to you and your experience. It can be a place you have actually visited or one that you imagine. The place does not have to be real, or even *possible*. You can be sitting on a big blue pillow floating on the surface of a quiet sea. You can be stretched out in a hammock suspended in space. You can be in a cave of clouds. Your special place must be one in which you can be alone and it must produce a positive feeling in you. It is in this special place that you will have an increased receptivity to further suggestions. That is, once a peaceful feeling is established, you will be responsive to imagery which reinforces and supports posthypnotic suggestion.

STEP 6. CONCLUDING THE INDUCTION
Enjoy your special place for another moment and then I will begin to count from one to ten and you can begin coming back to full consciousness, come back feeling refreshed as if you had a long rest. Begin to come back now. One . . . two . . . coming up, three . . . four . . . five . . . six . . . seven . . . eight . . . nine . . . and ten, open your eyes and come all the way back, feeling great. Very good.

Upon completion of the induction, a feeling of well-being should be suggested to avoid an abrupt return, which may cause drowsiness or a headache. You should feel relaxed and refreshed. You may walk around to make sure you are fully alert and congratulate yourself on doing a good job.

Recording the Complete Relaxation Induction

The six steps above have given you an overview of the *Relaxation Induction*. The steps described the general progression from an alert state into a deep trance. Now you are ready to use the induction in its entirety.

Before recording, you will need to do the following:

1. Read the induction aloud several times in order to become familiar and comfortable with its content. Review the preceding discussion of the hypnotic voice and apply that information to

your delivery of the induction. For the most part, say the induction slowly, keeping your voice level. You will need to experiment with tone and stress until you are satisfied with the way the induction sounds. You should be *convinced* when you hear yourself saying it. If you sound self-conscious, your tape will be, at best, minimally effective.

2. Time the length of your induction as you say it and compare it to the length of tape you will be using. You don't want to begin taping, only to find out that the tape you are planning to use is not the correct length.

3. When you are satisfied with the way your induction sounds and the length of time it will require, make sure that you have closed out any sounds that may be picked up by the tape, such as clocks, the television, the telephone, or the doorbell. You will also need to alert your family or roommates. Make sure they understand that you are not to be interrupted and they are not to make any sounds that can be heard in the location where you will be recording.

4. Put on comfortable clothing and get in a comfortable position. You may want to lie down, sit in a rocking chair, or sit at your desk with your feet up. Whatever your preferred position, make sure it is one that will be comfortable throughout the entire recording session. If you are shifting around or feeling physically uncomfortable, this discomfort will be reflected in the tone and quality of your voice.

5. Most important, perhaps, is for you to mentally prepare yourself to be relaxed and open so that your hypnosis will be effective. You cannot *make* hypnosis work by willing it to, any more than you can will yourself into sudden happiness from a state of despair. Whatever happens during your induction must be *allowed*, not forced.

THE RELAXATION INDUCTION

Because this induction will be used in later chapters that deal with specific hypnotic treatments, it is divided into two parts: *Going Down* and *Coming Up*. If you are using the induction solely for the purpose of relaxation, it should be recorded as one piece and not divided in any way.

Take a nice deep breath, close your eyes, and begin to relax. Just think about relaxing every muscle in your body from the top of your head to the tips of your toes. Just begin to relax. And begin to notice how very comfortable your body is beginning to feel. You are supported, so you can just let go and relax. Inhale and exhale. Notice your breathing; notice the rhythm of your breathing and relax your breathing for a moment. Be aware of normal sounds around you. These sounds are unimportant, discard them, whatever you hear from now on will only help to relax you. And as you exhale, release any tension, any stress from any part of your body, mind, and thought; just let that stress go. Just feel any stressful thoughts rushing through your mind, feel them begin to wind down, wind down, wind down, and relax. And begin with letting all the muscles in your face relax, especially your jaw; let your teeth part just a little bit and relax this area. This is a place where tension and stress gather so be sure and relax your jaw and feel that relaxation go into your temples and relax the muscles in your temples and as you think about relaxing these muscles they will relax. Feel them relax and as you relax you'll be able to just drift and float into a deeper and deeper level of total relaxation. You will continue to relax and now let all of the muscles in your forehead relax. Feel those muscles smooth, smooth and relaxed, and rest your eyes. Just imagine your eyelids feeling so comfortable, so heavy, so heavy, so relaxed and now let all of the muscles in the back of your neck and shoulders relax, feel a heavy, heavy weight being lifted off your shoulders and you feel relieved, lighter and more relaxed. And all of the muscles in the back of your neck and shoulders relax, and feel that soothing relaxation go down your back, down, down, down, to the lower part of your back, and those muscles let go and with every breath you inhale just feel your body drifting, floating, down deeper, down deeper, down deeper into total relaxation. Let your muscles go, relaxing more and more. Let all of the muscles in your shoulders, running down your arms to your fingertips, relax. And let your arms feel so heavy, so heavy, so heavy, so comfortable, so relaxed. You may have tingling in your fingertips. That's perfectly fine. You may have warmth in the palms of your hands, and that's fine. And you may feel that you can barely lift your arms, they are so relaxed, they are so heavy, so heavy, so relaxed. And now you inhale once again and relax your chest muscles. And now as you exhale, feel your stomach muscles relax. As you exhale, relax all of the muscles in your stomach, let them go, and all of the muscles in your legs, feel them relax and all the muscles in your legs, so completely

relaxed right to the tips of your toes. Notice how very comfortable your body feels, just drifting and floating, deeper, deeper, deeper relaxed. And as you are relaxing deeper and deeper, imagine a beautiful staircase. There are ten steps, and the steps lead you to a special and peaceful and beautiful place. In a moment you can begin to imagine taking a safe and gentle and easy step down, down, down on the staircase, leading you to a very peaceful, a very special place for you. You can imagine it to be any place you choose, perhaps you would enjoy a beach or ocean with clean, fresh air, or the mountains with a stream; any place is perfectly fine. In a moment I'm going to count backwards from ten to one and you can imagine taking the steps down and as you take each step, feel your body relax, more and more, feel it just drift down, down each step, and relax even deeper, ten, relax even deeper, nine . . . eight . . . seven . . . six . . . five . . . four . . . three . . . two . . . one . . . deeper, deeper, deeper, relaxed. And now imagine a peaceful and special place. You can imagine this special place and perhaps you can even feel it. You are in a [INSERT SPECIAL PLACE]. *You are alone and there is no one to disturb you. This is the most peaceful place in the world for you. Imagine yourself there and feel that sense of peace flow through you and sense of well-being and enjoy these positive feelings and keep them with you long after this session is completed, for the rest of this day and evening, tomorrow. Allow these positive feelings to grow stronger and stronger, feeling at peace with a sense of well-being, and each and every time that you choose to do this kind of relaxation you will be able to relax deeper and deeper. Regardless of the stress and tension that may surround your life, you may now remain more at peace, more calm, more relaxed, and allow the tension and stresses to bounce off and away from you, just bounce off and away from you. And these positive feelings will stay with you and grow stronger and stronger throughout the day as you continue to relax deeper and deeper.*

Enjoy your special place for another moment and then I will begin to count from one to ten and as I count from one to ten you can begin coming back to full consciousness, and will come back feeling refreshed as if you had a long rest. Come back feeling alert and relaxed. Begin to come back now. One . . . two . . . coming up, three . . . four . . . five . . . six . . . seven . . . eight . . . nine, begin to open your eyes, and ten, open your eyes and come all the way back, feeling great. Very good.

Using the Self-Guided Relaxation Induction

You may prefer to use a *Relaxation Induction* that is not taped. If so, change the *you* to *I* in the above induction and then silently lead yourself through, using basic key steps as your guide.

You will begin by thinking, "I will relax every muscle in my body, from the top of my head to the tip of my toes." After each key step you will think the phrase, "I feel my body drifting, floating, down deeper, down deeper, down deeper, into total relaxation."

Below is a list of the basic key steps you will use for your self-guided induction. It may help you to think of the induction as being composed of four major sections: (I) the head to chest section, consisting of steps 1 through 7; (II) the stomach to toes section, consisting of steps 8 through 10; (III) the special place and positive feelings section, consisting of steps 11 through 15; and (IV) the coming up section, consisting of steps 16 and 17.

The basic key steps are as follows:

SECTION I
1. Notice breathing, relax breathing.
2. Relax face, jaw.
3. Relax temples, eyes, eyelids.
4. Relax back of neck, shoulders.
5. Relax lower back.
6. Relax arms.
7. Relax chest.

SECTION II
8. Relax stomach.
9. Relax legs.
10. Relax toes.

SECTION III
11. *Going Down,* ten to one.
12. Imagine special place.
13. Imagine peace, sense of well-being.
14. Stress and tension bounce off and away.
15. Positive feelings will grow stronger.

SECTION IV
16. *Coming Up,* one to ten.
17. Feeling great.

It is important to note that the effectiveness of the self-guided induction, compared to that of the recorded induction, depends on you as an individual. You may want to try the induction both ways, as a recording and silently, to determine which type provides you with the most successful hypnotic experience.

3

Hypnotic Communication

Effective hypnotic communication is based on *suggestion*. Think, for a moment, about the ways in which various forms of suggestion play an integral part in your daily life. You get up in the morning and stumble over your son's jogging shoes, which have been abandoned in the hallway. As he approaches, your glance slides from the shoes to his gaze. The suggestion: Your shoes are not where they should be; move them. You drive to work, passing a billboard showing a group of euphoric people listing to KJOY. The suggestion: Your life will be happier, joyful even, if you listen to the same radio station these people listen to. Your employer enters your office, takes a seat, and says, "We're looking for someone to serve as project director and will be making a decision by the end of the month. We're extremely pleased with the way you have organized and implemented the training program. You've accomplished a great deal, and have the respect of your co-workers. How do you feel about the new project?" The suggestion is twofold: You are being considered as project director. And what can you say to sell yourself as the successful candidate? You stop by the bank on the way home, and the man in line behind you is smoking a cigar. The smoke is billowing into your face. You turn, look at the cigar in the man's hand, then make eye contact with him. The suggestion: Do something about the smoke for which you are responsible. You go out to dinner. After the entree, the waiter comes to your table and asks, "May I show you the dessert menu?" The suggestion: You are encouraged to order dessert. You come home and your 15-year-old daughter bounds out of her bedroom, greeting you with "Wouldn't you like to hear my report on the feeding habits of the bladdernose seal?" The suggestion: You would like to sit right down and listen to the report.

You will notice that these suggestions vary in their degree of directness. Further, some are verbal and some nonverbal. In hypnotic communication, you will be using both direct and indirect verbal suggestions.

The Hypnotic Suggestion

Technically, a suggestion is a proposition for belief or action that is accepted in the absence of intervening and critical thought. In other words, when you are hypnotized and in a relaxed state, your subconscious is more responsive to suggestion than it is when you are in a fully conscious state. The suggestion travels a direct channel to the subconscious, where it effortlessly becomes a belief, modifies behavior, or produces an effect or action.

Here are some of the objectives that can be achieved through the use of suggestion:

OBJECTIVE	SUGGESTION
To deepen a trance	*Relax and let your mind and body drift deeper into relaxation with every breath you take . . .*
To elicit a physical response	*Feel your arms grow heavier and heavier . . .*
To change emotions	*Feel your anger melt away . . .*
To alter behavior	*You are now a nonsmoker, you do not want to smoke . . .*
To create imagery	*Imagine yourself in a wide, green, peaceful meadow . . .*

Major Types of Suggestion

Described below are the six major types of suggestion: relaxation, deepening, direct, imagery, indirect, and posthypnotic.

1. Relaxation suggestions put you at ease, introduce a state of receptivity, and direct your focus inward while shutting out external conditions. These suggestions establish a comfortable foundation for further suggestions.

Begin to relax, just feel yourself relax deeper and deeper, and with every breath you take you find yourself relaxing deeper and deeper and becoming more responsive to positive suggestions.

Feel your muscles relax and feel your neck and shoulders relax, and as they relax you will find your mind relax. As your mind relaxes, you are more relaxed throughout your whole body and you are less and less aware of your environment.

2. Deepening suggestions take you into a deeper hypnotic trance. They provide an activity that has a single focus and intensifies your trance state in a number of ways. You can think of a deepening suggestion as a descending elevator — when a certain button is pushed, it goes down to the next floor. Three of the ways that suggestions can be deepened are illustrated below.

In a moment I am going to count backwards from ten to one, and you can imagine taking the steps down, and as you take each step feel your body relax, more and more, feel it just drift down, down each step, and relax even deeper, ten, relax even deeper, nine . . . eight . . . seven . . . six . . . five . . . four . . . three . . . two . . . one . . . deeper, deeper, relaxed.

Your eyelids are closed shut and they are so shut you cannot open them. They have been glued shut and are resting and you cannot open them. Your eyelids are tightly shut, very tightly shut and they are stuck together so tightly they will not open. You will count to three very slowly and you will think about your glued eyelids and when you say each number your eyelids will become more tightly closed. Try to open them . . . one . . . they will not open . . . two . . . they are closed shut . . . stuck shut, completely shut . . . three, your eyelids will not open.

You are so relaxed in your chair, your body is becoming one with the chair, you cannot move from the chair or get up or walk around, you are completely still in your chair like a statue. You are a statue resting in your chair. So relaxed in your chair that you cannot move. So relaxed that when you try to move your body will not move in the chair. As you try to move, your body is too relaxed to move in the chair.

3. Direct suggestions are designed to guide you or instruct you to respond in a certain way. Direct suggestions are usually simple and to the point. They are often used in an induction that does not require you to use your imagination to any significant degree. They are the opposite of indirect suggestions, in which imagery plays an integral part.

As direct suggestions are given, you respond to the words rather than the images. The suggestion may be one word or several sentences that trigger an immediate response. Some common direct suggestions follow:

Now you will go back in time to the scene that set the stage for your problem.

You feel drowsy, let the drowsiness come over you and let go of the images of the past.

Say yes to yourself and notice which finger wants to move and be your "yes" finger. When you feel a tug in your "yes" finger let it move. Now raise your "yes" finger when you know the date when you will begin to express yourself with confidence and self-assurance at work.

When I count to three you will be able to use your voice and you will describe the day your grandmother had her accident.

4. Imagery suggestions augment the other suggestions. They create mental pictures and set scenes that have specific purposes, such as to relax, to foster a new self-image, to serve as a "rehearsal" for new behavior, or to provide an environment in which any behavior can be reprogrammed. For example, the image of a stairway augments the countdown, a deepening suggestion. Images from your past augment your recall of an important incident, which is the result of a direct suggestion. Any kind of image or metaphor may be used with an indirect suggestion, such as an image of a strong, surging river to represent a person's circulatory system or of a singing bird to represent hope. Posthypnotic suggestions are expanded through the use of images as you imagine yourself successfully carrying out a new activity.

You feel you are as strong as the young man you were when you hit home runs on the sandlot. You can feel the bat in your hands, the excitement of being ready for the pitch. You feel the swing and the powerful connection you make with the ball, you watch the ball sail over the fence as you sprint easily from base to base. You have that same energy, that same euphoria and confidence all over again.

You go to your special place in the Arizona desert where, this time of year, the brilliant pink and copper sunsets stretch out for miles along the horizon, where the air is dry and clear, and there is silence all around you. Everything is so still, so silent, you can hear your own thoughts.

You are at the beach where your stress melts from you, slides down your body and is swept out to sea, just melts from you and washes away, and you stand without the weight of stress and you feel lighter and happier and are full of peace and of calm.

5. Indirect suggestions are of two major types. In the first, a desired emotional state, such as happiness, is focused on. The hypnotic subject is interviewed about his or her past and an experience is identified that once provoked the desired emotional state. Next, the subject is motivated, during the induction, to relive the experience and the positive emotion that accompanied it. A simple cue that can be used later to evoke the emotional state posthypnotically is then associated with the experience. For example, the subject may have recalled a particularly pleasant time in his youth when he was sailing with his father. He felt carefree, peaceful, and joyful. The subject reexperiences that event in the hypnotic state. He feels carefree and at ease. A cue word is introduced that can be associated with these positive emotions. The cue word is *sailing*. From then on, the subject needs only to think of the word *sailing* in order to experience the desired emotional state.

The second type of indirect suggestion is often associated with the work of Milton Erickson. Although he was not the first to use this technique, he certainly was the boldest and one of the most influential. Erickson used metaphors and analogies within the framework of hypnosis to give suggestions outside the conscious awareness of the subject. He sometimes used lengthy dialogue to put his subject into hypnosis, told stories, and presented analogies that the subject responded to and incorporated into his own behavior. The result was a change in the subject's experience, such as the elimination of chronic pain or a modification of a problematic behavior. For example, if Erickson were talking to a married couple who were not having successful or satisfying sexual relations, the problem would be approached metaphorically by talking about an elegant, satisfying dinner that is not consumed all at once, but is quietly and leisurely enjoyed.

The indirect suggestion is highly individualized. Each analogy, each metaphor, must fit the problem and the subject as closely as possible. For example, if an elderly man who had worked as a carpenter all of his life came to hypnotherapy to be relieved of pain in his arm, an induction would be designed to make use of a metaphor that was particularly meaningful to this man. The closer the metaphor could get to his experience, the better. For example, the induction might develop the image of an ironwood tree in order to stress the attributes of strength and wholeness associated with this wood. The induction might go as follows:

> *You are driving in the desert. The road is long and winds high above the desert floor. Suddenly, as you round a curve, you see an ironwood tree standing on a hill. One of the branches is being battered about in the wind . . .*

The hypnotherapist would then work within the metaphor to achieve a specific goal. In this case, of course, the goal would be to eliminate the pain the man was experiencing in his arm.

6. Posthypnotic suggestions are given during the induction and carried out upon completion of the induction, at a specific time during the posthypnotic phase. This type of suggestion is used to eliminate a habit, such as smoking, or to modify behavior in some other way, such as improving personal relations at work or increasing self-confidence. You hear the posthypnotic suggestion, incorporate it into your subconscious, reach full consciousness at the conclusion of the induction, and respond to the suggestion on a subconscious level at a later time. Here are examples of some common posthypnotic suggestions:

> *The next time you sit down to enjoy a meal, you will find yourself enjoying a smaller portion of food. You are full and satisfied with a smaller portion.*

> *As you begin your work day, you will feel more motivation than you ever felt before. You will make phone contacts and sales easily because you are confident, secure, and completely believe in the product you are selling.*

> *Upon completion of this induction, you will have totally lost the urge to smoke.*

> *Tomorrow you will walk into the examination room, sit down, take a deep breath and complete your exam feeling calm and relaxed and recalling easily and quickly all the correct information that you need.*

Guidelines for Effective Suggestions

There are some guidelines that should be carefully observed when you are formulating your own suggestions. Each of these will be discussed in the material that follows. Briefly, they are:

- Keep direct suggestions simple and concise.
- Repeat suggestions.
- Keep suggestions believable and desirable.
- Create a time frame for suggestions.
- Be certain that suggestions can be interpreted literally.
- Limit your suggestions to accomplishing one goal at a time.
- Break major goals down into a series of suggested incremental steps.
- Use words that are positive, rather than negative or discordant.
- Avoid relaxation suggestions that are thought-provoking.
- Use cue words or phrases to trigger and emphasize suggestions.
- Select appropriate images to augment direct and posthypnotic suggestions.
- Remove unwanted suggestions.

Keep direct suggestions simple and concise. When you are hypnotized, it is absolutely necessary for you to clearly and quickly understand what is being suggested. A direct suggestion should not be buried in a lengthy monologue. Many subjects respond to direct suggestions more effectively than they would to imagery. A person who cannot visualize *can* assimilate and act on a direct suggestion. Programming then takes place.

As illustrated below, a direct suggestion has a clear, single purpose, which is sharply focused.

When I count to three you will go back to the day you moved in with your foster parents.

You will shut out all the sounds around you. You will enjoy an inner silence.

Go back in time to the first experience you had in an airplane.

Repeat suggestions. Repetition is important because it helps you strengthen and retain the suggestion. As you repeatedly receive the same message, the suggestion becomes instinctive. You act on it automatically, readily, and with ease. Regardless of the nature of your specific suggestions, you can make it repetitious in one of three ways.

1. You can repeat it exactly: "You have stopped smoking, stopped smoking. You have stopped smoking."
2. You can paraphrase the key suggestion: "You have stopped smoking. You no longer want to smoke, you are not a smoker, you are a nonsmoker."
3. You can use synonyms or similar phrases to reinforce the same suggestion. Your purpose is to state the positive suggestion in many different ways in order to give it strength, to make it familiar, and to ultimately modify your behavior in some way.

If, for example, you are having difficulty concentrating on crucial exams, you might suggest:

You are <u>concentrating</u>, focused, <u>concerned</u> <u>only</u> with the exam in front of you.

This particular style of reinforcement is especially appropriate for use in the *Progressive Relaxation Induction* in Chapter 2:

You are completely <u>relaxed</u>, you feel <u>calm</u>, at <u>ease</u>, and <u>content</u>.

Keep suggestions believable and desirable. You need to think you can accomplish the objective of the suggestion and you must *want* to do it. If you don't believe you are capable of the change the suggestion proposes, then you are likely to reject it. Further, if you don't really want to pass the bar exam, lose weight, or be an effective public speaker, then your suggestion will be only superficial.

Create a time frame for suggestions. You do not need to set a rigid schedule of behavior modification for yourself, but you do need to indicate, within reasonable limits, the amount of time in which you expect something to occur. If you want to designate immediate action, use the words "now," "shortly," or "in a moment."

If the goal is to relax your shoulders, you could expect that to happen within minutes or seconds; in other words, immediately.

<u>Now</u> relax your shoulders, just let your shoulders relax. Feel your shoulders relax and <u>now</u> relax your arms, just let your arms relax.

A short time frame is also indicated in the following:

<u>Shortly</u> you will be able to recall the scene in your dream that made you so afraid; the scene will then be completely clear to you.

<u>In a moment</u> you will raise your finger to indicate that your hand is numb, that you have no feeling in your hand.

If your goal is a long-term effort, you may need to say, "By the time my classes begin," or "When I drive across the bridge next week, I will . . . ." It is necessary to be specific when using hypnosis with natural childbirth, as described in Chapter 8. You would say:

As you continue to relax, imagine the birth day arriving on . . . [INSERT THE APPROPRIATE TIME, BASED ON YOUR DUE DATE. FOR EXAMPLE, "six months from now," "September third," OR "tomorrow."]

It is particularly important to specify a time frame for activities such as studying, image rehearsal for athletes, or working on a creative product. Otherwise, a zealous subject could continue to work vigorously to the point of exhaustion. You might say:

Every morning you will work on your play. You will write with ease and inspiration. At noon you will stop and reflect on what you have done. You will review your work and feel a sense of accomplishment.

With a suggestion such as this you have the option to continue working in the afternoon or evening, but a stopping time is specified to keep the suggestion completely effective and realistic and to prevent exhaustion.

Be certain that suggestions can be interpreted literally. If you suggest to a field and track participant that he will "run like a deer" in his next competitive race, the runner conceivably could attempt to run on all fours.

The literal suggestion need not be that blatant to provoke an undesirable response. For example, in an actual case a hypnotherapist gave a woman the following suggestion:

Tonight you will leave your office, turn off the lights, and go home feeling relaxed and calm. When you get home, you will continue to feel relaxed and calm.

That evening, the woman left her office. *Then* she sought a way to turn off the lights, because her suggestion had been given to her in that order. She went outside, found the fuse box that controlled the lights throughout the building, and turned them off. The therapist, of course, had intended his client to turn off the office lights *as* she left her office, but that is not what he said.

There are two exceptions to this literal interpretation of suggestions. As mentioned in Chapter 1, if any suggestion is either personally harmful or in conflict with the subject's moral code, it will not be followed. You could not, for example, suggest that someone rob a bank and expect to have that suggestion followed unless the subject wanted to rob a bank and was merely waiting for permission to do so.

Limit suggestions to one problem area at a time. Trying to accomplish too many changes at one time or reprogram several areas of your life all at once will only dissipate the effect any one suggestion can have.

You would not, for example, try to stop smoking and lose weight at the same time. You would not try to eliminate insomnia and agoraphobia within the same two or three months. While it is conceivable that you could accomplish both objectives simultaneously, there is no need to overload yourself by shifting hypnotherapy into a miracle-working gear.

Major goals should be broken down into a series of suggested incremental steps. A suggestion can only be effective if it is directed toward an obtainable action or goal. It is necessary to examine your major problem and your final goal and than start by taking one minor modification within the problem area.

As you begin to experience a small amount of success from a suggestion, you will be motivated to increase that success. You may think of your suggestions as the rings on an archery target. You start at the outer ring and hit it; it's a small success. You then proceed to the next smaller ring, which is a suggestion slightly more difficult, and so forth, until you hit the target's center. This center represents the very core of the attitude, behavior, or problem you wish to modify or eliminate. For example, if you are trying to change your destructive, irrational behavior on the freeway, you might begin by not yelling at every person who pulls in front of you or, as you see it, "cuts you off." You than progress step-by-step until you can actually let someone else pull in front of you and smile while you're doing it because you realize that a less self-defeating behavior will make your commute less stressful. You will also come to recognize that being generous on the freeway will not, in the long run, make any difference in your commute time.

Remember that success tends to beget success. So keep your suggestion modest in the beginning and build on it, and the results will not only be rewarding, but also permanent.

Use words that are positive, rather than negative or discordant. It is necessary to use simple, brief, and direct statements when formulating suggestions. Avoid words such as *no, try, can't,* and *won't.* The subconscious reacts in accordance with positive affirmations such as *I can, I am,* and *I will.*

For practice in formulating positive suggestions, try the following exercise. On the lines at the left, write simple, single statements about the behavior that you intend to change in your life. Mention any habits you need to reduce or eliminate.

_____	_____
_____	_____
_____	_____

Now read over your statements and look for negative phrases, such as *I can't, I don't, I won't, I'll try.* (If you haven't used any negative words such as these, you are already thinking positively and should be able to easily envision your goals.) If you have used negative terms, rewrite your statements on the right side. This time, state your suggestions as if they had already been achieved. For example:

I don't want to be tense.	I am more relaxed.
I will try to lose weight.	I am losing weight.
I won't have another cigarette.	I am a nonsmoker.

Just as self-defeating as negative words are odd, discordant, or bizarre words that call up unpleasant images or muddle the intent of your suggestions. For example, this suggestion would be out of place during a *Relaxation Induction:*

> *Now jump from your neck to your shoulders and relax your shoulders...*

The use of the word *jump* in this case would be in opposition to your goal, which is to relax. If you were talking about relaxing your feet, you would not say:

> *Feel the relaxation winding its way around your left foot like a coil...*

You might then imagine your circulation being cut off, or a snake winding its way around your foot, or any number of other negative or confusing images.

Avoid relaxation suggestions that are thought-provoking. In the beginning stages of an induction, when relaxation is of major importance, keep suggestions general so that you may avoid thought-provoking responses. A typically safe relaxation suggestion would be:

> *Relax and drift and float into a comfortable state of relaxation. Just feel your whole body relax . . .*

An overly specific relaxation suggestion such as the following is undesirable because it is thought-provoking.

> *Relax and just imagine yourself as a child drifting and floating on a rubber raft on a lake. Remember how you felt as you drifted on the lake. Remember how relaxed you felt . . .*

If you once had a bad experience on a raft, or boat, if you cannot swim, or if you were afraid of being left alone as a child, this suggestion would cause a great amount of discomfort. Instead of relaxation, you would be likely to feel anxiety or even fear.

Use cue words or phrases to trigger and emphasize suggestions. Cue words are used in both posthypnotic suggestions and indirect suggestions. In posthypnotic suggestions, you will find the cues especially helpful if your goal involves habit control.

For example, the cue word for an overeater may be *full*. This triggers the suggestion given during the induction that whenever you feel the urge to snack during the day you will say the word *full* and no longer be in need of food.

Another cue word suggested during an induction session could help you maintain a normal blood pressure in the face of frequent attacks of stress and anxiety. On the freeway, in the midst of heavy traffic, you grow increasingly tense. Your palms begin to moisten and your stress level begins to rise. At this point you simply say your cue word quietly. It may be the word *open,* which is in direct contrast to feeling tense, "uptight," and anxious.

In an indirect suggestion, a cue word can be used to recall a specific emotion, time, and place. The word acts as a response button that takes you back to a time in the past when you felt a certain way that you now want to reexperience. For example, you may have once hiked in the Big Sur woods on weekends. You felt energetic, happy, and carefree. Your cue word, *Big Sur,* can be used to transport you to this time and place so that you can feel the emotion that was attached to the experience.

You may want to improve your relationship with your employer. Every time your boss talks to you, you find yourself feeling under stress. This results in negative, defensive, inappropriate behavior. Your cue phrase may be *shielded from stress.* When the boss calls you into his office, you say the cue phrase to yourself. This allows you to behave more positively, without defensive reactions to his requests, discussions, or observations.

Cue words provided important emotional support to a woman who had extremely low self-esteem and was enormously self-conscious about her appearance. She was given the cue word *Queen Elizabeth* to say to herself before entering a room in which she would have to interact with people. This cue suggested to her that she had self-worth and importance and should hold her head high. As she began to use the cue, her posture no longer betrayed her lack of confidence, and she was able to project a noticeable amount of self-esteem. With continued use of the cue, she began to feel increasingly better about herself because she was received and reacted to in accordance with her improved self-image. Her new expectations that people would react positively to her were met the majority of the time.

Select images to augment direct and posthypnotic suggestions. These images serve as a supportive framework as you reprogram yourself. *Each image should contribute to the achievement of your main objective.*

Your imagination has power, and a mental image can predict a real outcome. When you vividly imagine yourself reaching goals or improving various areas of your life, you actually activate certain brain activities and types of energy that help you reach your goals. Imagination can also set up failure. If you imagine yourself not being able to bike up that hill, or pass that exam, you probably won't.

Athletes successfully use a "mental workout" by imagining themselves strengthening their abilities, increasing the speed of their performance, and winning. Writers and artists use imagery to motivate their production. Students use imagery to pass exams. They imagine themselves taking an exam while feeling relaxed and focused and passing with flying colors. Public speakers imagine speaking in front of a group, enjoying the speech, feeling calm, relaxed, and appreciated.

Earlier in this chapter, you did an exercise that required the use of positive suggestions. Now you can practice strengthening those suggestions by making them more explicit and more stimulating. You will do this by creating positive imagery.

Fold a piece of paper into halves, vertically. In the left column, state your goal in a positive way. (This is your posthypnotic suggestion.) In the right column, create a positive image that indicates how you will *feel, look,* and *be* when you have reached your goal. Here are two examples:

POSTHYPNOTIC SUGGESTION	POSITIVE IMAGERY
I am more relaxed at work.	I am sitting at my desk next to the window. It is a pleasant, sunny day. I am calm and at ease. My work is in front of me and is progressing well.

I am losing weight.	I look in the mirror and see that I am much slimmer and trimmer. I go into my room, reach into my closet and take out my old size ten skirt, try it on, and it fits perfectly. I feel proud of myself and physically attractive.

The more vivid and clearly defined an image is, the more effective it will be. You can intensify a positive image by incorporating all of your senses—smell, touch, sight, hearing and taste —into it. The more you can use your senses, the more real the image will seem to your subconscious.

For example, in a *Relaxation Induction,* you could establish a sense of peacefulness with the following example of guided imagery. Or you could use the same image to provide the setting of your special place, the place where your posthypnotic suggestion will be made.

SIGHT	Imagine a *beautiful beach* with *white sand* that *stretches as far as you can see,* and a *dazzling blue sky;* you
SOUND	can *hear the pounding of the surf, children laughing in the distance* and the *sound of seagulls crying* and as
TOUCH	you walk along the beach you can *feel the coarse sand giving way beneath your feet* and the *warmth of the sun on your shoulders.* And now you take a deep breath
SMELL	and *smell the freshness of the ocean air.* You
TASTE	*taste the salt,* the *cool moisture* that catches in your lungs.

Remove unwanted suggestions. These may be suggestions that are included to test suggestibility or to emphasize imagery. For example, the Balloon Test is used to gauge suggestibility. In this exercise, the subject is told that a number of helium-filled balloons are tied to his or her wrist. The balloons rise and pull the wrist and arm upward, floating higher and higher into the air. At the end of the test, the subject is told that the string and balloons have been removed from the wrist, and the wrist and arm have returned to a normal position. If these unwanted suggestions are not removed, the subject may experience the arm lifting and floating again at a later date.

A university professor was given the suggestion that she was a passenger on a bus. It was raining, and the motion of the bus and the sound of the rain were lulling her into a relaxed and sleepy state. As she gazed out the front window of the bus, her attention was caught by the rhythmic motion of the windshield wipers. (At this point a metronome began to tick rhythmically, and it was suggested that the sound of the ticking was the sound of the windshield wipers ticking back and forth.) As she watched the wipers, she felt sleepy and drowsy and soon entered a deep trance.

The subject responded quickly and easily to these suggestions. However, the ticking of the metronome and the motion of the windshield wipers were not removed. A few days later the subject found herself driving her car in the rain, on her way to the university. She turned on her windshield wipers and started to feel drowsy. Fortunately, the subject knew what she was responding to and simply removed the unwanted suggestion herself.

To safeguard against any unwanted suggestions that may be left in an induction, you can simply suggest, "You will return to normal and reject all suggestions that are not related to the areas of self-improvement."

Evaluating Suggestions

Each of the following ten suggestions is incorrect in some way. It has not been constructed in accordance with the information covered in this chapter. Read each suggestion and find its flaw; then describe it briefly on the lines below.

1. *The noise outside does not disturb you. It does not disturb you in any way . . .*

_____

_____

2. *At the count of three you will go back in time to the first time you were frightened by a dog. You will recall it and on the count of six you will recall the second time you were frightened by a dog and you will remember how you felt and what you saw and then you will . . .*

_____

_____

3. *Relax and just imagine yourself swinging in a swing, imagine that you are eight years old and your brother is pushing you as you swing. Relax and just think about that time . . .*

_____

_____

4. *Relaxation is oozing through your body. It is hopping from your head to your feet.*

_____

_____

5. *The sun is so hot, so bright, and so hot . . .*

_____

_____

6. *You see yourself as slim and trim. You have lost weight.
   Now you will come back to full consciousness as I count
   from one to ten.*

_____

_____

7. *As you begin to study, you are totally absorbed in your
   work. You forget all about the time and concentrate completely on what you are learning . . .*

_____

_____

8. *In traffic you become so calm, so relaxed and calm, you
   concentrate on the car in front of you. You close out all
   the other bothersome traffic . . .*

_____

_____

9. *You will stop smoking, stop smoking, stop smoking. You
   will also find yourself satisfied with smaller amounts of
   food and you will not have the need to eat between meals.*

_____

_____

10. *You are trying to go up the hill on your bicycle and your
    legs push hard against the pedals. You finally make it to
    the top.*

_____

_____

11. *Imagine yourself in your special place. You are in your
    special place and you like it there. It is pretty, and you
    feel comfortable.*

_____

_____

12. *The music in the background is the signal for you to relax.
    You relax when you hear this music and you feel as if
    you could easily sleep. You will have no trouble sleeping,
    the music is your signal to sleep. Now you will come
    back to full consciousness when I count from one to ten.*

_____

_____

Now take a look at the flaws which were "planted" in each example and check to see how many of them you correctly identified.

1. *Noise* is a discordant word; *not* is a negative word. A better wording would be "The sounds will only help you to relax."
2. This direct suggestion is not simple and concise. It requires too much from the subject. It should read: "At the count of three you will go back in time to the first time you were frightened by a dog."
3. This is a thought-provoking "relaxation" exercise which is likely to produce the opposite result. The subject may be afraid of heights, may have once fallen from a swing, or may not like his or her brother.
4. *Oozing* is a word which may cause you to conjure up inappropriate images. *Hopping* is a discordant word; relaxation would not hop. *Flow* would be a more effective word to use in both sentences.
5. You could interpret this suggestion literally and grow uncomfortably warm.
6. The suggestion needs to be reinforced by repeating the statement, paraphrasing the statement, or using synonyms: "You are slim and trim, you feel light, you like feeling slim and trim, you feel better now that you are thinner, much better."
7. A time limit should be set. If not, you may continue to study until exhaustion takes over. You could suggest, "You will study in the afternoon, working successfully, until four o'clock when it is time to rest and reflect on what you have learned."
8. This is a dangerous suggestion to interpret literally. Rather than the directive to concentrate on the car ahead, there should be a cue word that signals a calm state without limiting your driving abilities.
9. Two goals are embodied within this suggestion. It attempts too much and will be ineffective.

10. *Trying* and *finally* are negative words. You are not accomplishing the goal with ease. It is a struggle; therefore, the image is not positive.
11. Imagery should be used to augment the direct suggestion. "Imagine yourself in your special place, the moon is out and you can smell the pine trees, hear the creek washing over the rocks, it is completely peaceful, the air is still and fragrant, and you are peaceful . . ."
12. You need to remove the suggestion that this particular piece of music will put the person in a sleepy state. The subject may hear the music while driving, shopping in a supermarket, watching a movie, attending a party, or another place where sleeping would be inappropriate or even dangerous.

The Success Equation

You now have all the relevant information regarding types of inductions, specific suggestions, and the entire general hypnotic presentation. But there is one tremendously important key component that has thus far gone unexamined. It is *belief*. Without this component, successful hypnotic communication is impossible. You must have belief for the process to work.

Three factors operate with belief: *imagination, motivation,* and *anticipation*. If you can imagine something and it is within reasonable limits, you will be quite likely to achieve it. Studies have proven that as an activity is vividly imagined the body's internal system reacts in exactly the same way it would if the activity were actually being performed. Neurons fire in the same pattern, and small contractions occur in the muscles involved in the imagined activity.

This kind of imagining is a form of practice. To engage in it, you first need to pinpoint exactly what you want to achieve. Then you imagine that you are doing the task, performing the skill, engaging in the activity with complete success. You should also imagine yourself experiencing the rewards from your success.

For example, if your goal is to finish your master's thesis, you see yourself actually researching, writing, and submitting the thesis. You see the whole process from sitting at a table in the library to walking in the professor's door to submit your thesis. You see the color and feel the texture of the binding on your manuscript. You feel the weight of it in your hand as you carry it and set it down on the desk. Then you imagine the rewards. These may include high praise from a specific faculty member, the publication of your thesis, or invitations to speak on your selected subject area.

If your goal is to sell more real estate, you see yourself interviewing the clients, showing the house, writing the contract, making the offer, completing the sale, filling out all the necessary forms, and receiving your commission. As a reward, you may see yourself cashing the commission check and buying a present for someone—even for yourself.

Athletes use this type of practice, called *image rehearsal,* to improve their skills. They actually imagine each part of the athletic event as if it were occurring. For example, a baseball player would imagine the sound of the crowd, the smell of the ballpark, the brightness of the lights on the field, the feel of the bat in his hands, the pitcher winding up, the color of the pitcher's uniform, the calls from the crowd. He would imagine his swing, a perfect one, feel the bat connecting with the ball, and watch the ball sail into the bleachers as he heads for first base.

When this type of image rehearsal is practiced on a regular basis, it results in the production of a highly developed physical and mental energy which increases *motivation.* Thus, you have the first part of the equation: *imagination* × *motivation* = *belief* in yourself.

Taking the equation one step further leads us to *anticipation.* Anticipation occurs when your subconscious is thoroughly convinced that you are capable of your goal.

Think, for a moment, about a comedian. He expects the audience to laugh. He anticipates that they will. The audience in turn expects that he will entertain them. He comes onstage, both anticipations match, and the audience laughs. This illustrates a fundamental principle of human behavior: People behave in the ways that they are expected to behave.

If you expect your employer to respond favorably to your suggestion, he is more likely to do so than if you did not expect him to. If you anticipate increased sales in the next month, sales are quite likely to rise.

An excellent example of this anticipatory phenomenon is the story of the three women who often go gambling together. They enter the Las Vegas casino, arrange a time to meet at the door late in the evening, and each go their separate ways. At the appointed hour they reconvene at the main door, and the first question asked is never "Did you win or lose?" The question they invariably ask each other is "How much did you win?" The fact is that all three women *do* win 90 percent of the time.

Imagine that a male subject is about to meet someone for the first time. The person he is going to meet may be a blind date, a prospective employer, his new in-laws, or a public figure he has long admired. Regardless of who it is, the person's reaction is important to him and he is very anxious for the person to like him. However, he convinces himself that the person will not like him for one reason or another. He even goes so far as to imagine the person being disappointed when he or she sees him. He may anticipate being totally ignored. Entering into a situation while exhibiting this type of anticipatory behavior will most likely produce very disappointing results. This man's expectations will be fulfilled.

The major flaw here, of course, is that the man did not first imagine positively, become motivated, and then believe so that he could anticipate in a positive way. So now you have the whole equation: *Imagination × motivation = belief + anticipation.*

Guided Imagery Suggestions: A Supplement

As explained in the guided imagery section of Chapter 2, your special place can be any place you like. It can be a location you recall from a past experience or it can be a place you have made up; it does not even have to be *possible.* As you use guided imagery, keep these guidelines in mind:

1. If you are using a location from a past experience, make sure that you do not associate even the slightest negative feeling with it.
2. The more intensely you can imagine your scene, the more successful your suggestion will be.
3. The most important components of the scene are peacefulness and solitude.
4. Be inside the scene, experiencing it firsthand. Don't stand at a distance, viewing yourself as if you were in a movie.
5. After you have experienced your suggestion fully, bring yourself out of the place and back up to full consciousness.

You may want to use one or two of the following four guided imagery selections as they are, or you may want to revise one to meet your own personal preferences. They are included here as a quick reference and to give you an idea of the various possibilities that exist for developing your own individualized imagery.

THE LAKE

You are lying on a wooden dock, resting comfortably on a thick exercise mat. The dock extends out into a clear, blue lake that is bordered by tall, fragrant pine trees. The water slaps gently against the dock pilings. The sky is radiantly blue and bright and shimmering as if it were a band of silk stretching across the sky above your head. A few clouds dissolve and float like pale feathers high above you. You lie very still and feel a slight breeze against your cheek. You hear only

*the sound of your own breathing and the constant lapping motion
of the water. Then you close your eyes and feel the delicate warmth
of the sun on your eyelids, your cheeks, your hair, your neck, and your
whole body. You feel completely serene and relaxed, completely relaxed.
You are so relaxed you can imagine reaching your goal . . .*
[ENTER POSTHYPNOTIC SUGGESTION.]

PATH IN THE WOODS

*Close your eyes and make sure you are comfortable. You are about
to take a leisurely walk along a path that leads you into a lush forest,
safe and secure. As you walk along this path your legs stretch out with
every step, relaxing all of the muscles in your legs; and as you walk
along, your arms are comfortable and you breathe deeply and easily. Every breath relaxes you more and more, and off in the distance
you can hear the sounds of birds chirping and the rustle of the leaves
as a breeze flows through the tops of the trees. As you walk along the
path, you hear the sound of water splashing from a stream nearby,
and soon you come upon this stream and find a comfortable place
to stop and relax even more. Water has trickled from the stream into
shallow rocks, forming a still, crystal-clear pond. You kneel on the
grass and look into this pond to see a wonderful, positive reflection
of yourself. You are smiling and happy. You are looking as good as
you feel, and you feel wonderful inside and out. You dip your hand
into the clear water and take a sip. The water is cool and refreshing.
You look into the pond again, and the water becomes still. You can
see your goals, see yourself reaching them in the most positive way . . .*
[ENTER POSTHYPNOTIC SUGGESTION.]

A ROOM IN THE COUNTRY

*It is a mild summer day. You are in your favorite comfortable clothes,
sitting in the second floor room of an old country inn. The inn is built
of wood and stone, and your private room is spacious, with polished
hardwood floors and a large, comfortable bed. You have brought some
things with you. These are on the table. You look at each one . . .* [IN-
SERT THE POSSESSIONS YOU WOULD LIKE TO HAVE WITH YOU—A CERTAIN
PHOTOGRAPH, A BOOK YOU WANT TO READ, A BOTTLE OF YOUR FAVORITE WINE, YOUR
NEW CAMERA.] *You sit in a large, comfortable chair, put your feet up,
and gaze out your window over the rolling, grassy hills. A hedge of
wild blackberry bushes winds its way in a crooked line over the
horizon. All around the inn it is quiet, very quiet, and no one else
is here to disturb you. One lone blackbird swoops in easily over the
crest of the hill, the air is clear and fresh and filled with the faint scent
of wildflowers. You can look out the window as long as you like. You
feel your body relax all over as you gaze from the window. Your heart-*

beat slows a little, you breathe easily, your mind is free of any worries you have about your family, your job, or yourself. All your cares melt away. No one is going to ask you for anything, or expect anything of you. You are free to do anything you please, your mind is relaxed. And because you are so relaxed you can imagine reaching your goal . . . [ENTER POSTHYPNOTIC SUGGESTION.]

ROCKING

You are sitting in a rocking chair on a beach at the edge of the sea, but you are not near enough to get wet, and when the water rushes in it stops a few yards from you, slips under itself, and back out again. You rock easily with the rhythm of the sea, and as you rock you watch each wave, and each wave takes away another care. It slips in and washes away a care, taking it out to sea where it disappears in the depth of the water. And you rock slowly and the sea washes your cares away, one by one, and your mind is free and you feel as if you could rock here forever. You are completely relaxed and because you are so relaxed you can imagine reaching your goal . . . [ENTER POSTHYPNOTIC SUGGESTION.]

4

Weight Loss

How many times have you chosen one of a possible hundred diets and followed it rigidly until you lost weight? You suffered, your stomach growled, and all you thought about was that you *could* have the four ounces of carrot juice, but you *couldn't* get within twenty yards of a french fry. You may have accepted this agony as an inevitable part of the weight loss process.

Then, finally, you reached your goal. You even lost five extra pounds to give yourself some leeway. You thought you could stop your diet and eat normally, so you did, and in a few weeks you had gained all of that old weight back again. This is a familiar, almost monotonous, tale. But it illustrates the most prevalent factor in unsuccessful weight reduction: The loss of pounds is not permanent when you restrict food from your body without considering the causes of overeating.

Notice that this chapter addresses those people whose weight is a result of overeating. It does *not* address those whose obesity is the result of physiological causes. Studies have shown that there is no proof that overweight people are "more neurotic" as a group than those whose weight is average or below. While there are standard psychological causes for overeating, this does not mean that all overweight people overeat. Many, in fact, have been found to eat less than people who were underweight.

If, then, you do fall into the category of overweight overeaters, your problem is not in your metabolic rate; it is, most likely, in your mind—your subconscious mind. You may have lost weight with lots of conscious effort. Your conscious mind served as a military force to keep your hunger habits from invading. But, as soon as you reached your goal and stopped dieting, your subconscious took over again. This is because the subconscious is a great deal stronger than the conscious mind, and you did what you were most strongly directed to do: You ate more than your body physically needed.

While the subconscious is no simple power to grapple with, it is only through permanent changes in this part of your mind that you will experience permanent changes in your life—changes that come automatically and are not painful. If you can accept the subconscious as your friend, instead of your enemy, you will be able to take a look at what is causing behavior that, ultimately, makes you unhappy.

Shaking Hands With Your Subconscious

The reason you overeat may not be at all clear to you. That is, you may not recognize the culprit if it walks right up and sits down at the dinner table with you. And why is this so? Any motive that is capable of making you operate in a way that causes you long-term physical, emotional, social, or mental discomfort is a motive that has, most likely, been well buried in order to avoid recognition. Excavating the reason will not be as difficult as you may suppose, because there are only a few major causes. The following are the most common reasons anyone, including you, may overeat.

You eat to reward or entertain yourself. From the very beginning of your life you have been rewarded with food for your accomplishments—anything from a simple task to a monumental success. Look, for example, at a "chronology" of food rewards in a lifetime. As a baby you get a cookie as a reward for picking up your toys, saying "please" or "thank you," or responding to "potty training." As a growing child you get dessert for cleaning your plate, or at least for eating your brussel sprouts, and you get cookies for practicing your cello. Your teacher gives a candy to each student who gets an A on the spelling test. When you are a teen-ager, the coach takes your team out for pizza after a good game. You go to the movies to be entertained, and you further entertain yourself by consuming a soft drink, popcorn, and a bar of candy. When you graduate, your parents take you out to the best restaurant they can afford.

When you're an adult, you get promoted to sales manager, and you celebrate by going out to dinner. You take prospective clients out to lunch. You go on a much-needed vacation with your overworked, neglected body, and the first thing you do is seek out those great little restaurant "finds."

You may be reading this and thinking, "A lot of these examples fit me, or come fairly close, but the trouble is that I *enjoy* these activities. And how can I avoid these situations if I really want to? If I need to participate in a breakfast meeting with our biggest client, how can I get out of it? What can I say?"

You don't need to say anything. You can go to the breakfast with new habits firmly established in your friendly subconscious. In fact, you can go to *any* food-focused function and still enjoy being there.

You eat to lessen or negate an unpleasant experience. Again, the pattern is established when you are very young. You are teething and miserable, so you get a tasty teething biscuit, the perfect antidote for sore gums. Then you fall off your playswing. As the well-meaning adult is drying your tears, you get a cookie. The pattern continues throughout your life. You don't get accepted to the college you applied to, so you go out and binge with your friends. You lose that important contract, so you plop down in front of your TV set (which accepts you whether or not you set the world on fire) and gulp down a few goodies. You go out with someone you really like, the date doesn't go well, and you *know* you'll never see the person again. You walk into the kitchen and find yourself a little comfort in the contents of your refrigerator.

You can add to these examples. You know which things are so upsetting that they propel you to that cute little bistro around the corner where the fondue is delicious. But how long does the consumption of food negate the earlier unpleasant experience, such as losing the contract? If you are honest, you will probably have to admit that the hurt is only partially desensitized while you are devouring the cheesecake. But if you had a time schedule to show how long the food *acts* to buoy your feelings, as opposed to how long you *wear* the food, it would be easier for your rational self to take over.

You eat because you want to be noticed, to gain authority. You can have a very big body and, at the same time, an exceptionally small ego. You may need to command more attention, feel more important, actually take up more space than those around you. If this notion seems far-fetched, consider the amount of attention you give to any individual who is tremendously overweight—someone you squeeze past in the aisle at the supermarket, someone who wedges himself in the seat in front of you at a play, who overflows the seat adjoining yours in the airplane. There is a certain fascination with an individual of great size. Even though the fascination is often negative, it is, at least, some form of attention. Most people would probably agree that in any area of life it is far easier to get negative attention than positive attention. With very little effort, this kind of casual and momentary notice can be provoked.

You eat when you need love. This statement is a difficult one to make. Try, for example, substituting "I" for "you." Say, "I eat when I need love." The declaration almost hurts. The more uncomfortable you feel trying this one on for size, the more likely it is to be the cause of your overeating—and it is a perfectly logical cause. Go back to the beginning of your life again. As a baby, you cried and you got a bottle. If you were lucky, you got *held* and had a bottle at the same time.

Now you eat when what you really want is to have someone smile at you, give you a kind word, touch you, give you a hug. You may want someone to make love to you, so you love yourself by giving yourself lots of wonderful things to eat. The trouble is that this behavior creates a treacherous cycle: As you create a bigger self, the more likely it is that your self will be, from a social point of view, unlovable. Unfortunately, our society rewards thin and scorns fat, which leads us to the next major cause.

You eat because you are afraid. Afraid of what? There are more than a few possibilities. One common fear is of the potential of your own sexuality. If you are unattractive to the opposite sex, you do not have to worry about the consequences, problems, opportunities, and decisions a relationship can bring. You can stay in your present situation, which demands nothing of you emotionally or physically, because you are not sought after.

One woman artist feels so strongly about her work that she allows herself to get "up in pounds," as she puts it, because "I don't want to be physically attractive. I don't want to have to worry about it. Men don't seek me out and I don't have to deal with a relationship. I can devote myself to my work."

You may be thinking that there are talented, interesting, and overweight people who still have sexual appeal, and, of course, this is true. But the general rule is that you are not enticing, nor do you seem receptive, if your attractive self is literally buried.

For this reason, a husband may encourage his wife to stop for donuts or a hot fudge sundae when he knows that her resistance is low, that she has just arduously taken off three pounds and will rapidly gain it back again if she follows his suggestion. Why does he do it? It is his insurance against her attracting male attention and finding that she has options, and his finding that he has competition. This last factor serves to increase his insecurity, which was the reason he tried to insure the safety of the relationship to begin with.

Another fear may be related to good health. You may have been raised to believe that thin was unhealthy and therefore undesirable. The message you received as you grew may have been "If you are plump, you are healthy. If you are healthy, you are less vulnerable to disease." So you make sure that you always have pounds to spare and thus keep illness at bay.

Where Do You Go From Here?

Regardless of the cause of your overeating, the procedure you follow for change will be the same. You need to replace the emotional satisfaction that food provides with an activity that serves the same purpose. For example, during a busy day you may need to stop and take a break. A snack is just the thing to help you relax, but what you really need at this moment is an appealing, satisfying alternative. A good alternative to snacking would not be to clean your windows or drive to the bank. It would be to sit down, close your eyes, relax for five minutes, and listen to some soothing music.

One male writer achieved a successful and permanent weight loss when he replaced his usual snack with jogging six city blocks whenever he needed a change in activity or a relaxer. When he returned from his short bout of exercise, he was genuinely not hungry. He had renewed energy and a clearer mind and went back to work refreshed.

Pinpointing When, Where, and Why You Eat

The following exercise will help you to further analyze your eating pattern. To identify when you are most likely to eat, where you eat, and why you eat, check a yes or no next to each item in the list below.

WHEN		Yes	No
I eat when I am	hungry	———	———
	nervous	———	———
	bored	———	———
	stressed	———	———
	hyperactive	———	———
	happy	———	———
	sad	———	———
	lonely	———	———
	frustrated	———	———
	anxious	———	———
	afraid	———	———
	other:_____	———	
	_____	———	

WHERE		Yes	No
I eat too much or snack	while watching TV	____	____
	in groups	____	____
	while reading	____	____
	during coffee breaks	____	____
	between office/home	____	____
	at sports events	____	____
	at business lunches	____	____
	at social events	____	____
	in bed	____	____
	other:_____	____	
	_____	____	

WHY		Yes	No
I treat myself to a snack or meal whenever I need	love	____	____
	reward	____	____
	companionship	____	____
	something to do	____	____
	a change in my activity	____	____
	to compensate for something unpleasant	____	____
	to relax	____	____
	to feel more important	____	____
	to feel secure	____	____
	sexual attention	____	____

After you have pinpointed the times, locations, and reasons you overeat, you can begin to change your behavior pattern. Look back at the WHEN category. Which ones are marked "Yes"? In the chart below, under the WHEN heading, write, "I eat when I am (nervous, bored, and so on)." Follow the same procedure for the WHERE and WHY categories. Now you should have three or more statements that ring true for you. (If they don't, go back and review your checks. Find the ones that have been incorrectly placed.)

WHEN   NEW OPTIONS:

_____   _____

_____   _____

_____   _____

_____   _____

WHERE

_____   _____

_____   _____

_____   _____

_____   _____

WHY

_____   _____

_____   _____

_____   _____

_____   _____

Now look at the right hand column marked NEW OPTIONS. Don't fill this in immediately. Give yourself plenty of time to think of alternative activities. Make sure that these activities genuinely appeal to you. They are ones that you will commit yourself to during hypnosis. You need to be able to stand behind them. Below is an example of substitute activities—new options—for old habits.

WHEN	NEW OPTIONS
I eat when I am bored.	When I am bored, I read a newspaper, a magazine, or a book. I call a friend, go for a bike ride, go to a movie.
I eat when I am nervous.	When I am nervous I take five minutes to close my eyes and relax. I jog in place, participate in some other form of physical exercise, or work on my current favorite project or hobby.
I eat when I am lonely.	When I am lonely I telephone a friend, write a letter, run an errand for someone who needs assistance, or interact with my older neighbor who needs company.

WHERE

I eat too much or snack between the office and my home.	On my way home from work I go for a drive to a scenic spot, take a walk, shop, stop at the racquet club and swim.
I eat in bed.	When I am in bed I will review my accomplishments and good qualities before going to sleep. I will read, or make a schedule for the next day.

WHY

I treat myself to a snack or meal whenever I need a change in activity.	If I am engaged in a sedentary activity such as sitting at my desk, I change to one which is mobile, such as doing sit-ups. If I am engaged in an activity which is mobile, I change to one which is sedentary, such as reading.

Setting Up Your Plan of a Lifetime

Now that your problem is written out before you and you have established your options, you need to look at your overall objectives. These are the same from person to person, regardless of the specific details of your weight problem. They are:

1. To experience weight loss
2. To maintain weight loss
3. To incorporate new habits into your life

The third objective is really the key to numbers 1 and 2. As you already know, the amount you eat and the way in which you use food is a pattern that has been established in your subconscious. In order to change your negative eating pattern, a new pattern must be created. *You need to reprogram your subconscious.* This is accomplished through self-hypnosis.

Reprogramming for Results

The *Weight Control Induction* in this chapter is designed to help you think, feel, and act in certain ways. The induction reprograms your subconscious by offering logical and realistic suggestions. Below are the specific objectives necessary to achieve weight loss, maintain weight loss, and incorporate new habits. You need to:

Give less importance to food as it relates to your feeling of well-being. The induction suggests, "I eat the correct and reasonable amounts and I am totally satisfied. I am satisfied from one meal to the next." And later, "I am relaxed and peaceful and food is less and less important."

Build up your confidence and self-esteem so you can accept a slimmer self. The induction suggests, "I reflect on all the positive things in my life, the goals and successes I have already achieved, and I know that I will continue to be successful, reaching every goal that I have, and creating the most healthy and positive life for myself. And now I imagine seeing myself, stomach flat, hips and thighs firm and trim, legs firm and slim. I look great and feel so good."

Increase the appeal of healthful foods. Make them more desirable and make fatty foods less desirable. The induction suggests, "And now I imagine for a moment a table, a table in front of me, and I fill this table with foods that are harmful to me, foods that are harmful to my body and emotions. They are like poison to my system. If I choose to eat any of these foods, I eat a small, small amount, a very minute amount of these foods satisfies me completely. So now I push these foods off that table, push them away from me. And now on that empty table I place the many foods that I enjoy anyway. Good healthful foods, foods that contain fewer calories, such as _____." You will finish the sentence by inserting the names of the low calorie foods you most enjoy.

Incorporate into your life new patterns of behavior in regard to times, places, and reasons for overeating. The induction suggests, "I now have new ways of dealing with my old habits." At this point in the induction you will insert the statements you listed earlier in the NEW OPTIONS column. "When I am _____, I _____." Be sure to include a new option for each condition you have listed in the WHEN, WHERE, and WHY column. You will see exactly where to place your new options in the induction which follows.

The Total Induction

Now that you understand the way the induction works, you are ready to use it. The *Weight Control Induction* is used with the *Relaxation Induction* in Chapter 2. You may remember that the *Relaxation Induction* was divided into two parts. The *Weight Control Induction* comes *between* the two parts. The three components should not be separated from each other as they are used or taped; instead they should blend into each other in one continuous flow. Keeping that in mind, follow this procedure:

1. Turn to Chapter 2 and use the *Going Down Induction.*

2. Use the *Weight Control Induction* that follows.

3. Turn to Chapter 2 and use the *Coming Up Induction.*

WEIGHT CONTROL INDUCTION

Because you are now at peace and relaxed, you can be successful at reaching any goal, at losing weight. You are imagining that you have lost the amount of weight you no longer want or need and that you have maintained that weight loss. You imagine and feel and think of yourself as slimmer, slimmer, thinner, thinner, muscles tight, total body in shape. Your unconscious will now act on this image and realize and actualize this image. And you will allow yourself to lose weight, to lose weight, lose the amount of weight you no longer want or need and to maintain that weight loss.

You change negative eating patterns into good patterns now. You allow this to take place easily and effortlessly. And now you imagine for a moment a table, a table in front of you, and you fill this table with foods that are harmful to you, foods that are harmful to your body and emotions. You imagine these foods; they are sweets, snack foods and junk foods. You place them on the table. These foods are all harmful to you. They are like poison to your system. These kinds of foods cause you to gain weight you no longer want or need. If you choose to eat any of these foods, you eat a small, small amount, a very minute amount of these foods satisfies you completely and that satisfies you completely. You couldn't eat another bite. So now you push these foods off the table, push them away from you, your body rejects these foods. Your mind and emotions reject these foods. You clear the table. And now on that empty table, you place the many foods that you enjoy anyway. Good healthful foods, foods that contain fewer calories, such as _____. [INSERT THE NAMES OF LOW CALORIE FOODS YOU MOST ENJOY.] *There are the fruits that you enjoy: cool, clean, and crisp. There are the vegetables you enjoy. You see those good, healthful foods on that table, and you imagine eating those good foods. And you eat slowly, eat slowly. Whether you are conversing or not, you are totally aware of the amount you are eating, and you eat modest portions and then stop, and that feels fine, and that feels fine. You eat correct and reasonable amounts, and you are totally satisfied, and you are totally satisfied. You are satisfied from one meal to the next and have no desire to snack between meals.*

You feel totally proud of yourself. You reflect on all the positive things in your life, the goals and successes you have already achieved, and you know that you will continue to be successful, reaching every goal that you have, and creating the most healthy and positive life for yourself. And now you imagine seeing yourself, stomach flat, hips and thighs firm and trim, legs firm and slim. You look great and feel so good. You are relaxed and peaceful, and food is less and less important, and you are more comfortable eating more slowly. Snacking is unimportant to you, regardless of where you are, or what you are working on, at home or at work. You can eat small amounts of food in a restaurant, and you will eat more slowly. You may leave part of your meal on your plate, and that is fine.

Regardless of stress, you are more at peace and relaxed, and food is less important to you. You feel proud of yourself. The rewards are tremendous. And now whenever you think of eating, you choose those good healthful foods. And you eat the correct amount. And when you have eaten the correct amount you stop eating, you stop eating. You stop eating. You may even leave some food on your plate, and that is just fine. You simply stop eating. And continue to relax. And allow that sense of confidence now and peace now to flow through you. You are more motivated now than ever before to create the most healthy and positive life for yourself, to change old eating patterns into good eating patterns, to lose the amount of weight you no longer want or need, and to maintain this weight loss.

You now have new ways of dealing with your old habits. [INSERT ALL OF YOUR WRITTEN STATEMENTS FROM THE NEW OPTIONS COLUMN CHANGING I TO you.] *These new habits will make permanent weight loss possible.*

You feel wonderful, and you can begin to experience a new and healthy vital energy that flows through your body and mind. And your thoughts are positive, confident. You reflect on all of the positive aspects about yourself, your intelligence and creativity. And you see yourself as the attractive person that you are. And you allow these positive feelings to grow stronger and stronger for you every day, every night. And now you continue to relax.

What to Expect and Following Up

On completion of the induction, you should have begun to accept a slimmer self and to desire foods that contain fewer calories. In addition, you should have begun to establish new habits for when, where, and why you eat. Though your behavior should change immediately, your actual weight loss, of course, will be gradual. Regardless of the success of the induction, you cannot drop five pounds overnight.

Continue to do the induction every day until your desired weight loss is achieved. You may want to schedule the self-hypnosis at a regular time each day in order to experience consistent reinforcement.

For maintenance, use the induction once a week, or once every other week, as seems necessary.

Case History

Sally Marcos, a 42-year-old teacher, is five feet four inches tall and weighed 215 pounds at the time she began self-hypnosis. She had tried several popular weight loss programs in the preceding years. Her experience had been that she would lose up to 50 or 60 pounds, only to gain it back again within a few months. Hypnosis was her last attempt at maintaining weight loss.

After her first session, she noticed a change in her habits. Her hypnosis sessions continued on a weekly basis for four months, and her weight loss occurred at the rate of 2 to 4 pounds per week. Even though the reduction would occasionally level off, Sally eventually lost 100 pounds.

She continued to use self-hypnosis for six months. After she stopped, she gained back 20 pounds, but leveled off at an attractive 135. Because stress was identified as the major cause of her unhealthy eating pattern, she now uses the induction whenever outside pressures begin to escalate.

Special Considerations

As you use self-hypnosis to achieve weight control, remember to (1) determine your weight loss goal with consideration for your age and your bodily structure, and (2) allow yourself to lose weight gradually. Don't become impatient or have unrealistic expectations. The comforting general rule is that the more *gradual* the weight loss is, the easier it is for it to be permanent.

In rare cases, a person's weight gain will not be the product of overeating. There will be, instead, some physiological cause other than caloric intake. This cause may be an abnormal retention of water, low thyroid, or the use of a drug that disturbs the body chemistry. If you are one of these cases, you will recognize symptoms such as puffiness (as a result of water-retention) or general lack of energy (as a result of low thyroid). If there is doubt in your mind about your reason for being overweight, it is best to have your doubt dispelled or confirmed by a medical examination.

5

Nonsmoking

Tom Loffler, a third-year law student, gets out of bed in the morning, does fifty push-ups, eats a quick breakfast with his wife, and leaves on his bike for the university. He has not varied this routine for three years.

Ruth Navarette, a 60-year-old nonfiction writer, wakes at 5:00 A.M., brews a pot of French roast, collects the *Chronicle* from her front lawn, and returns to bed to read the paper and savor her coffee. She has done this every morning for as long as she can remember.

Lauren Holm, a single 45-year-old English professor, never sits down to dinner without bringing with him a necessary companion, his current reading material. (If, for some reason, Lauren is deprived of his book, article, or newspaper, he will compulsively read the catsup labels and sugar packets.)

Before Lisa McMasters goes to sleep, she rehearses the general plan for the day ahead. Lisa has done this every night since she became assistant program director for a local television station. Sometimes she reaches over to her nightstand for a piece of paper and jots down a few notes. With that concrete agenda to look forward to in the morning, she settles into sleep.

Rita and Jack Wiston, real estate agents in their mid-50s, light up their first cigarettes on their commute each morning. From then on, it's a cigarette every half hour for Jack and at least a pack-and-a-half a day for Rita. In twenty years of married life, this pattern has remained unchanged.

Each of these people, and millions of others like them, has a habit that is so well-ingrained it almost seems to be a reflexive action. Regardless of what the particular habit is, each has its own unique *satisfaction*.

Tom Loffler will feel energized by his push-ups. After an hour of early morning self-indulgence, Ruth Navarette will be geared to a day of self-motivated productivity. As Lauren reads, he will be transported by the printed word to a world that is more stimulating than his own. Lisa will feel comforted by her list of planned activities for the next day. And, of course, Rita and Jack Wiston will experience a temporary lift every time they light up.

Taking away any one of these habits would cause personal distress and create severe disruption. Each of them seems permanent. And if you're a smoker, you *know* how permanent a habit can seem to be. You may have forgotten the original reason you began your habit, or perhaps you just found yourself smoking one day, without any apparent reason. Though you now want to end the habit, you have always felt that stopping was next to impossible. All the medical data and scare tactics in the world can't seem to influence you to quit. And the reason for this is simple: The habit has not been established by the logical, intellectual part of your mind; instead, the habit's cause lies in your subconscious. If you want to change your behavior, you must first recognize the reason or reasons you smoke. Below are the key reasons anyone smokes.

You smoke to nurture yourself. You wake up in the morning feeling a bit dull, and your work day looms before you with no reward in sight. You light up and get a quick lift, a slight elevation of mood, and feel better prepared for your day.

Or maybe you're home alone most of the time. You feel cut off from interaction with the outside world. You may even feel ignored. The companionship of your cigarettes lessens those feelings of isolation and loneliness. If your children have just gone off to college, or you are experiencing some sort of separation or transition in your life, your dependency on these "friends" becomes even stronger. In the absence of any other support group, they are there.

You smoke to relieve stress or provide a break in your activity. The pressure at work builds all day. There does not seem to be a way for you to let off steam or to seek calm territory, so you have a cigarette. The act of stopping what you are doing, lighting up and inhaling deeply, does several things. (1) The cigarette allows you to take a miniscule physical break from whatever you may be doing—from computer programming to leading museum tours to styling hair. If you are actually lighting a cigarette, you cannot be expected to be doing something else at that same moment. (2) Taking a deep breath to inhale the cigarette is, in itself, a relaxing exercise. (As you have learned, breathing deeply is part of the *Relaxation Induction*.) (3) If only for an instant, smoking puts you in an anticipatory frame of mind. When you light up, you look forward to a few moments of pleasure. Stress is briefly put away as you renew your spirit and bolster yourself to continue the activity which has caused the stress.

You smoke because you find social situations uncomfortable. You feel awkward with other people whom you do not know well. You don't know what to say to them, and you don't know what to do with your hands as you attempt conversation. You feel alone, a floater in a room of people, so you use the cigarette as a prop for your hands or even as a kind of anchor for making you feel more secure in social situations in which you would otherwise be very ill-at-ease.

At a party, cigarettes can serve as a kind of bond, pulling you into a group of smokers as you offer or accept a cigarette. You may use smoking as a vehicle for meeting other people, as your shared habit provides the opportunity for some safe, ice-breaking dialogue.

Finally, your self-image may be enhanced because you feel that smoking makes you appear more worldly, more confident and outgoing. You may have a lot of admiration for someone who smokes, and duplicating the other person's habit allows you some form of identification with him or her.

You smoke to control your weight. Cigarettes do suppress the appetite. You may be using your habit to try to take the edge off a normal appetite, or to control another habit—overeating. If you have a cigarette and coffee for breakfast, a cup of soup and two cigarettes for lunch, then you can enjoy a larger dinner—even if you can't really taste it.

Meeting the Need While Dismissing the Habit

Think about the above reasons. Each of them has a *positive* function; that is, it isn't wrong to be nurtured, to feel less stressed, to feel comfortable in social situations, or to control your weight. What you are accomplishing with cigarettes has value. It's just that the habit that has been established to meet the need is one that ultimately destroys, rather than supports.

You know there is nothing that can be said about the ill effects of cigarettes that you have not already heard more than once. Further, the suggestion that you can meet the same needs while employing a new behavior or a new habit may seem outright preposterous. But it isn't, if you're willing to rely on the power of your subconscious. Your subconscious can provide you with specific, constructive alternatives to smoking that will be genuinely desirable.

Pinpointing When, Where, and Why You Smoke

The following exercise will help you to analyze your smoking pattern. To identify *when* you are most likely to smoke, *where* you smoke, and *why* you smoke, check a yes or no next to each item in the list below:

WHEN		Yes	No
I smoke when I am feeling	lonely	_____	_____
	isolated	_____	_____
	ignored	_____	_____
	unhappy	_____	_____
	stressed	_____	_____
	insecure	_____	_____
	awkward	_____	_____
	uncomfortable	_____	_____
	unimportant	_____	_____
	other:_____		
	_____		

WHERE		Yes	No
I smoke too much	in the car	_____	_____
	in front of the TV	_____	_____
	at meals or after meals	_____	_____
	at my desk	_____	_____
	in the employees' lounge	_____	_____
	as I commute	_____	_____
	in a cocktail lounge or bar	_____	_____
	at social events	_____	_____
	other:_____		
	_____		

WHY		Yes	No
I smoke whenever I need	companionship	_____	_____
	a break in the routine	_____	_____
	comfort	_____	_____
	relaxation	_____	_____
	to control my desire for food	_____	_____
	to be noticed	_____	_____
	to look occupied	_____	_____
	other:_____		
	_____		

After you have pinpointed the times, locations, and reasons you smoke, you can begin to change your behavior pattern. Look back at the WHEN category. Which ones are marked "Yes?" In the chart below, under the WHEN heading, write, "I smoke when I am feeling (isolated, stressed, uncomfortable, and so on)." Follow the same procedure for the WHERE and WHY categories. Now you should have three or more statements that ring true for you. (If they don't, review the items and find the ones that you have marked incorrectly.)

WHEN	NEW OPTIONS
_____	_____
_____	_____
_____	_____
_____	_____
_____	_____

WHERE	
_____	_____
_____	_____
_____	_____
_____	_____
_____	_____

WHY

_____	_____
_____	_____
_____	_____
_____	_____
_____	_____

Now look at the right hand column marked NEW OPTIONS. Don't fill this in immediately. Give yourself plenty of time to think of alternative activities. Make sure these activities genuinely appeal to you. Since they are the ones that you will commit yourself to during hypnosis, you need to be able to stand behind them.

The following is an example of substitute activities — NEW OPTIONS — for old habits.

WHEN

I smoke when I am feeling isolated.

NEW OPTIONS

When I feel isolated, I visit a friend, make a telephone call, write a letter, offer to do something for someone else, read a newspaper, magazine, or book.

I smoke when I am feeling stressed.

When I feel stressed, I close my eyes and breathe deeply ten times; I go for a walk, talk to someone about what is causing the immediate stress, shift my attention to a constructive activity that I enjoy.

WHERE

I smoke too much while driving.

While driving, I breathe deeply and relax, concentrate on tightening and relaxing my muscles, plan my next activity in detail (a board meeting, a report, a dinner for guests, a phone call, a date).

I smoke too much while at social events.

At social events I join the nonsmokers, make a concerted effort to introduce myself to at least one unfamiliar person, and carry on a short conversation. I participate in discussions whenever the opportunity presents itself.

WHY

I smoke whenever I need a break in my routine.

If I need a break in my routine and I am engaged in a mental activity, such as writing a report, I change to physical activity, such as stretching, getting up and chatting with someone; getting some tea or water. If I am engaged in a physical activity, I change to one which is mental, such as thinking through plans for my next vacation, formulating a new and interesting facet in the area of my job which most interests me, writing a letter to someone I care for.

I smoke whenever I need to control my desire for food.	To control my desire for food, I cut out junk foods, reduce my intake of other high calorie foods, and eat fruits or vegetables for snacks.

Setting Up Your Smoke-Free Plan

You have now developed a concrete set of new options. Check over your list and make sure that every one of your options is as specific as it can be, and confirm within yourself that you are willing to commit yourself to it. These options all contribute to your two major objectives, which are to:

Become a permanent nonsmoker. It is absolutely crucial for you to see yourself as a nonsmoker. A nonsmoker is a person who *chooses* not to smoke. You do not see yourself as an ex-smoker, a person who *forces* himself not to smoke.

Incorporate new habits into your life. These new habits are itemized in your NEW OPTIONS chart.

As you know, the need for your habit has been established in your subconscious. It is your subconscious that causes you to nurture and support yourself by smoking. In order to be able to genuinely desire an alternative to smoking, you need to reprogram your subconscious.

Reprogramming for Results

Reprogramming is accomplished through a hypnotic induction that is especially designed to help you meet your specific needs and to alleviate the demands created by your daily environment. You need to:

Build confidence in achieving your goal. The induction suggests, "Reflect for a moment on all of the success you have already had in the past, the many positive goals that you have already reached and achieved, and feel proud, proud of yourself, proud of all the positive aspects of your life. Know without a doubt that because you have been successful in the past and because you have reached so many positive goals, you will continue to reach every goal that you have, will continue to be successful in every area of your life . . ."

Perceive cigarettes as being unappealing and distasteful. The induction suggests, "The smell of cigarettes is now disgusting and the taste is unappealing and unappetizing. Your mouth is clear of smoke, without any trace of cigarette taste, and it feels fresh. Your taste buds experience the appetizing, fresh tastes of your food."

Perceive yourself as a healthy, energetic person. The induction suggests, "There are no poisonous and unhealthy fumes circulating in your system. You now choose to be healthy, to be strong, to breathe clean air with your lungs clean and fresh. The less you smoke, the better you feel. Soon you will begin to notice that every aspect of your life begins to improve more and more. You will breathe more easily and regain a new, healthy and vital energy."

See yourself as a nonsmoker. The induction suggests, "You have all the right reasons to be a nonsmoker. You now make a conscious choice not to smoke that cigarette and emotionally you feel just fine. There is a smile on your face. You are a nonsmoker and it feels wonderful. You have stopped smoking cigarettes. See yourself in social situations, see yourself in any situation, enjoying yourself, feeling great without a cigarette, and that feels fine."

Incorporate into your life new patterns of behavior in regard to times, places, and reasons for smoking. The induction suggests, "You now have new ways of dealing with your old habits." At this point in the induction, you will insert the statements you listed in the NEW OPTIONS column in this chapter. If your induction is to be recorded, you will change the word *I* to *you.* (For example, "When *you* are driving *you* will breathe deeply ten times to relax.")

Include a NEW OPTION for each condition you have listed in the WHEN, WHERE, and WHY columns. Note that you do not try to use *all* the NEW OPTIONS at once. Begin by using one for each category (WHEN, WHERE, and WHY). Once these three options have become habits, you may insert your other NEW OPTIONS into the induction. The idea is to not overload yourself with new patterns of behavior. Introduce the patterns a few at a time. You will see exactly where to place your NEW OPTIONS in the induction that follows.

The Total Induction

Now that you understand how the induction works, you are ready to use it. The *Nonsmoking Induction* is used with the *Relaxation Induction* in Chapter 2. You may remember that the *Relaxation Induction* was divided into two parts. The *Nonsmoking Induction* comes *between* the two parts. The three components should not be separated from one another as they are used or taped; instead, they should blend into one another in a continuous flow. Keeping that in mind, follow this procedure:

1. Turn to Chapter 2. Use the *Going Down Induction*.

2. *Use the Nonsmoking Induction* that follows.

3. Turn to Chapter 2. Use the *Coming Up Induction*.

NONSMOKING INDUCTION

And as you are relaxing deeper and deeper, reflect for a moment on all of the success you have already had in the past, the many positive goals that you have already reached and achieved, and feel proud, proud of yourself, proud of all the positive aspects of your life, your creativity, your intelligence. Feel proud of yourself. And know without a doubt that because you have been successful in the past and because you have reached so many positive goals, you will continue to be successful in every area of your life, in every area of your life. You are now more motivated and more determined than ever before to reject all that is unhealthy and harmful to you: bad habits, tension, stress, the habit of smoking cigarettes. You now reject this habit of smoking cigarettes. You have all the right reasons to be a nonsmoker. You do it for yourself, for your health and well-being and that feels fine, that feels fine. And since you have been successful in the past, you will simply continue to be successful and reach every positive goal that you have, and you now choose to be a nonsmoker. You begin to feel and see an image of yourself without a cigarette or a pack near you. See yourself as a nonsmoker, you are a nonsmoker and that feels fine. You reject the habit of smoking, your mind rejects it and your body rejects it. Imagine throwing a pack of cigarettes out the window and away from you, and that feels great. You have made up your mind, you have made the choice to be a nonsmoker and that feels fine, it feels fine. Your body now rejects smoking cigarettes, your lungs no longer want those poisonous fumes in them. They now want to become clean and clear and healthy once again. Your sinuses want to feel clean, fresh air. The smell of cigarettes is now disgusting, and the taste is unappealing and unappetizing. Your mouth is clear of smoke, without any trace of cigarette taste, and it feels fresh. Your taste buds experience the appetizing fresh tastes of your food. There are no poisonous and unhealthy fumes in your system. You now choose to be healthy, to be strong, to breathe clean air with your lungs clean and fresh. You have all the right reasons to be a nonsmoker. And you have made up your mind and are now more motivated than ever to continue to create the most healthy, the most healthy and positive life for yourself, and you are now a nonsmoker. You feel it within. You now make a conscious choice not to smoke that cigarette and emotionally you feel just fine, feel just fine. You are a nonsmoker, a nonsmoker, and a positive feeling will stay with you throughout the day, wherever you go. Imagine your daily routine, what you would normally be doing, and see yourself doing these routines all without a cigarette, and feeling fine. You now have new ways of dealing with your old habits. [INSERT YOUR NEW OPTIONS, CHANGING I TO you, SUCH AS, "When you are at social events you will join the nonsmokers and start a conversation with someone you have not met before."] *This is a new way to deal with an old habit, and it is a successful way. It works and you feel fine, just fine. Imagine your daily routine without a cigarette and there is a smile on your face and you feel just fine. Whatever your destination may be, see yourself going there in your usual manner without a cigarette, breathing clean, fresh air, enjoying, enjoying being a nonsmoker. Continue to see yourself go through the routine of your day, feeling calm, feeling as calm and relaxed as you feel right now. There is a smile on your face. You are a nonsmoker and it feels wonderful. You have stopped smoking cigarettes. You consciously decide not to have that cigarette, and your emotions are fine, you feel just fine. It feels fine being a nonsmoker. Imagine yourself going through a typical day without a cigarette and it feels great. The less you smoke, the better you feel. Soon you will begin to notice that every aspect of your life begins to improve more and more, every day and every night. You will breathe more easily and regain a new and healthy vital energy. You are a nonsmoker and that feels fine. You are a nonsmoker and that feels fine. See yourself in situations, see yourself in any situation, enjoying yourself, feeling great without a cigarette, and that feels fine.*

What to Expect and Following Up

The length of time it takes to experience results from this hypnotic induction will differ according to the individual. Some people stop smoking after the first session, while others experience a complete cessation after repeated inductions for six months. After you have achieved the state of nonsmoker, you may later experience the urge to smoke again. If you do, begin to use the *Nonsmoking Induction* immediately. Don't let the condition build until the habit has become embedded in your subconscious again.

Case History

Bob and Louise are a couple in their fifties. Because Louise suffered from emphysema, it was imperative that she stop smoking. Bob supported his wife's effort to rid herself of the habit, and he decided to stop also. Both had smoked for many years and had often tried to stop, but failed. Each of them smoked five packs a day. If either of them left a cigarette burning in the ashtray, the other would finish it. Their habit seemed hopelessly well-ingrained. They had never experienced hypnosis. The induction and suggestions that were used were similar to the ones used in this chapter. Bob stopped smoking completely after the first session. Louise cut down to four or five cigarettes a day the first week. The following week she was able to quit completely. To date, a year has passed and the couple are still nonsmokers.

Special Considerations

Though most people do not have any trouble accepting an induction which reprograms the habit all at once ("cold turkey"), there are a few individuals who may not want to attempt this technique, fearing that it is too drastic for their subconscious to accept. If this is the case with you, an alternative is possible. You may use the same *Nonsmoking Induction* in this chapter, but instead of using the key statement, "You are now a nonsmoker," you may substitute "You are now smoking less than you did before." Then later, "You are now smoking much less than you did last week." Continue with this gradual affirmation until you reach the state of nonsmoking. Reword the suggestions throughout the induction to reflect a gradual change, rather than a total change.

During the same period of time you are using hypnosis, provide yourself with an environment that is as stress-free and nurturing as possible. You are bringing about a big change in your life, and anything you can do to reinforce your new behavior will make the transition easier.

6

Stress Reduction

Imagine a symphony orchestra that is beginning to get out of control. One violinist is three bars ahead of the rest of the string section. The percussionist is six bars ahead of the erring violinist, and the conductor has begun waving his arms in a tempo that is twice that of the score. The musicians perpetuate this chaos until the music escalates into a virtual frenzy. Finally, the members of this unfortunate orchestra collapse in a heap on the stage floor, their instruments strewn about them like implements of battle.

Similarly, as a person perpetuates stress and continues to endure excessive tension, he may experience an escalating frenzy or become a candidate for stress-related illness.

While certain types of stress can be good for you—such as the stress caused by a romantic encounter or the anticipation of a reward —stress that begins to debilitate or produce depression is completely undesirable. Such a condition calls for change. And while you may not be able to change the world, you can change your reaction to it.

First, examine the general cause or causes of your stress reaction. Literally hundreds of factors can cause stress—from noise to resentment, from fatigue to emotional upsets. Though the cause of your stress may seem evasive or even puzzling, it will no doubt fall into one of the major categories examined in the material below.

You have inherited a proclivity for stress. You learned how to show affection (or how *not* to show affection) from your parents. You learned certain public behavior by watching one or both of your parents in social situations. You learned your grandmother's recipe for spaghetti sauce by watching her make it. And you learned that certain situations most often produce, at least in your home, certain predictable patterns of behavior.

Your mother may have consistently shown stress whenever she was expected to entertain outsiders. Your liberal brother may have exhibited extreme stress whenever he discussed politics with your conservative father. The rest of the family may have felt stress whenever your brother and father were in the same room. These are extreme examples, but they illustrate the ways stress patterns exist within any family unit.

If your father always exhibited stress while driving, you got the message at an early age that driving was a stimulus likely to cause stress. As a result, driving may be a major situation that causes stress in you.

Your stress is inherited. You have learned to behave in the same way as someone you admired or depended on. This is called "modeling." Just as fears often "run in the family," so also do stressful reactions.

Additionally, stress that has been transferred from parent to child is sometimes intensified by the inherent physical makeup of the individual. Two children may both exhibit stress when exposed to the same stimulus—a noisy environment, for example—but one child may react to it more severely because of individual inborn differences.

You experience stress because you have a Type A personality. The definition of a Type A individual fits you if you are:

- Prone to overachievement
- In the habit of forcing yourself to work toward unrealistic goals
- Consistently competitive
- Constantly aware of time and prone to rushing
- Quick to exhibit anger
- Cynical

This list may seem to characterize a dismal individual, one who is hopelessly anchored in undesirable behavior. However, some of the most interesting people you know may fit into this category and *seem* to function quite successfully. What may not be evident is the core of the Type A's problem. He or she is *addicted* to stress. The stress constitutes a lifestyle and acts as a precursor of illness, as has been shown by recent studies linking Type A personalities and heart attacks. The hostility factor coupled with cynicism are the two key elements that make this group more susceptible than others.

You experience stress because of fears, awfulizing, and "shoulds." Focusing on the nightmares of life or *catastrophizing*, worrying about the worst possible alternative, can produce continual stress.

If you catastrophize or awfulize, you expect some form of disaster or danger at every turn. If your sister's husband and your neighbor's husband leave their wives to marry younger women with whom they work, you figure it is only a matter of time before your husband extends his office hours. If your sales are down for the month of September, you see yourself going out of business by the end of the year. If your 14-year-old daughter tells you she is in love with a freshman classmate, you see her burdened by two unwanted babies by the time she is 16. When you experience any pain or discomfort, it is magnified. A benign cyst is a deadly tumor, indigestion is food poisoning, a regular evaluation process by your employer forecasts the loss of your job.

Shoulds are nearly as disruptive to your emotional well-being. Shoulds consist of the rules you believe that you and others must live by. The trouble is, you make these rules up yourself. Then you try to follow them as if they are laws, and when you can't or don't, you feel as if you are a bad, disgusting, inferior person. You punish yourself with condemnation.

Here are a few of the shoulds that commonly plague people.

- I should be the perfect lover, friend, parent, teacher, student, or spouse.
- I should not make mistakes.
- I should look attractive.
- I should keep my emotions "under control" and not feel anger, jealousy, or depression.
- I should not complain.
- I should not depend on others, but take care of myself.

You probably have some of your own favorite shoulds you could add to this list. Unfortunately, your shoulds not only prevent you from having an accurate perception of yourself, but of others as well. You think that the people you know *should* behave according to your list of rules, and if they do not, they are willfully disobedient, uncaring, lazy, sloppy, stupid, or lacking in compassion and love. Living with this invisible list of burdens is unnecessarily debilitating.

You may experience stress because of inescapable pain or discomfort. This stress results from a real physical cause, such as chronic pain. Accompanying the physical sensations are ones of an emotional nature. When you experience any chronic disorder, it is also common for you to begin to feel "set apart" or isolated. You may feel searing guilt or anger for always being the "one who suffers," and eventually you may feel extremely depressed by your helplessness in the situation.

You experience stress because you repress and refuse to accept important feelings such as hurt, anger, or sadness. Some people try to entirely deny any negative emotion, viewing such responses as if they were the very root of self-destruction. These people will go to great lengths to keep from acknowledging their true feelings. They may demand constant attention, talk nonstop, overeat, drink excessively, exhibit defensive behavior, or turn everything into a problem. If the negative emotion is instead acknowledged and experienced, its intensity and duration are reduced.

Assume for a moment that you lose someone close to you through death. Your sadness is accompanied by depression. But you give yourself permission to mourn and put aside life for awhile. You reflect upon the past and evaluate the future. You sort out your feelings, rearrange them, and feel sorry for yourself. While you are doing this, other energies and emotions are allowed to rest. Even though you may not realize it, your mourning is releasing a major cause of stress that could, if repressed, become an influential factor in your life.

As a further example, imagine that a husband is irritated by his wife's devotion to her career and her careful attention to job-related plans, procedures, and details. At first, the husband is merely annoyed and doesn't exhibit any frustration. Next, he begins to feel as if her job is in direct competition with him. Then, finally, he decides—still without revealing his feelings overtly—that he is definitely number two and his wife's job is number one. At home, he continually feels under stress. Every phone call is an outside threat to his private life. Every business meeting his wife attends seems to be a pleasurable outing for her from which he is excluded. Instead of facing up to his perception of what is happening to his marriage and discussing his feelings with his wife, he allows his hurt to accumulate and intensify. This produces an extremely stressful situation that constitutes a domestic volcano, ever-ready to erupt.

You experience stress because you are exposed to a specific incident or particular stimulus that taxes your physical abilities or your mental or emotional capabilities beyond their limits. Think of a stressful experience, or a stress-stimulus, as a "prescription" that comes to you with the expectation that you fill it. You see its expectation as a demand, but you feel that you don't have the mental, emotional, or physical ingredients to fill the prescription.

It may be some portion of your job that stands unfilled at the prescription counter. It may be a part of your marriage that is not functioning effectively. Perhaps other's expectations for your attention or affection seem too high.

Your stress may have several combined causes. When examined individually, they seem insignificant; yet, if they occur all at once, they seem monumental. You may have started your day with a car that did *not* start for fifteen minutes. Just when you thought you were going to have to find another mode of transportation, the engine turned over. When you reached your office, you found that your secretary had not finished photocopying the status report that you were scheduled to present at a nine o'clock meeting. Then the lunch date you had scheduled with a prospective investor was canceled without reason, and your afternoon routine was interrupted by requests and calls that seemed, for the most part, trivial. When you returned home, your son told you he needed a ride to basketball practice (back through the commuter traffic from which you had just escaped). Your husband's plane was more than an hour late arriving, and by the time you both pulled up in front of a local restaurant for dinner, you felt as if you were a time bomb. This kind of day which seems so annoying and unavoidably stressful can be significantly modified by hypnotherapy. You will see how reprogramming prevents the minor irritations of the day from having a cumulative effect.

You experience stress because you have a dietary deficiency. Certain foods may cause your emotions to soar one minute and hit bottom the next. Sugar, caffeine, and alcohol are closely associated with stress. A lack of Vitamin B complex greatly contributes to irritability. The foods high in B complex vitamins are found in whole grains, brewer's yeast, liver, and legumes. If you are under severe pressure and you have poor eating habits or a "hit and miss" system for balancing your diet, the stress that you would normally feel will be magnified. It is not easy to determine which comes first—the dietary deficiency or the stress—because stress causes the depletion of B complex vitamins and the lack of B complex produces stress. In either case, hypnotherapy can work in conjunction with a new dietary plan to relieve or reduce stress. As you meet your nutritional needs, the *Stress Reduction Induction* will work as a major aid.

If you are female, you may experience stress as a product of PMS. Current estimates show that 33 to 50 percent of American women between the ages of 18 and 45 experience Premenstrual Syndrome. This amounts to between ten to fifteen million women. The physical and emotional symptoms of PMS commonly show themselves seven to fourteen days prior to the onset of the menstrual period. The physical symptoms include sugar or salt craving, fatigue, headaches, weight gain, bloating, and breast tenderness. The emotional symptoms include anxiety, confusion, temporary memory loss, and mood swings from euphoria to despair. Here again, proper nutrition can be a great help, and the addition of B complex vitamins can ease the symptoms. When dietary programs are used along with hypnotherapy, PMS can be greatly reduced, if not eliminated entirely.

Your Stress Assessment

In order for hypnotherapy to effectively cope with stress, the *Stress Reduction Induction* must be tailored to fit each person's specific needs.

These needs are determined by pinpointing the individual's stress stimuli and accompanying responses.

Chris is a 35-year-old divorced father who has permanent custody of his five-year-old daughter, Jana. Jana's mother is remarried, lives outside the U.S., and does not see her daughter. Chris's stress assessment will give you an idea of the scope of physical and emotional responses that can accompany various stimuli.

STRESS STIMULI	PHYSICAL AND EMOTIONAL RESPONSES
1. Jana asks why her mother won't come back.	Slightly light-headed, feeling of weakness, impulse to change the subject and repress emotion.
2. Having to review the inferior work, or discuss the inferior performance of an employee.	Tightness in chest, a lack of control over facial muscles, fear that I will give away my true feelings which are contempt for the employee's low performance, a feeling of resentment at having to deal with the problem.
3. The constant clatter Jana and her playmates make as they play in her room.	Muscles tighten, I grow quiet and feel invaded by outside forces and guilty about being upset.
4. Riding with a loud, abrasive co-worker who is a member of the company group commuter program and an erratic driver.	Flushed face, am afraid my anger will be evident, feel victimized, grow fidgety, and imagine telling him off.

Chris's case is a good example of how closely stress is linked with repression. Look at stimulus 1. Chris wanted to change the subject with his daughter because the conversation was too unpleasant. In stimulus 2, he can't express his feelings to his employee, so he resents the whole situation. In stimulus 3, he doesn't say anything because he feels guilty. His rational self recognizes his daughter's need to participate in play activity. In stimulus 4, Chris holds in his anger throughout the whole commute.

Chris examined his negative responses and developed positive responses to use in reaction to the same stress stimuli. (You will notice that stimulus 4 required a complete physical change, since the co-worker's driving was actually a physical threat.) Below are Chris's new, positive responses.

NEW RESPONSES

1. When Jana asks about her mother, I will relax, accept my feelings, show Jana affection, and talk about her feelings.

2. When I review the poor work of an employee, I will see myself as a guide, a person who has the opportunity to help someone else achieve a better work performance.

3. When Jana and her friends play, I will see the noise as healthy, happy outbursts and not feel that the noise will harm me in any way.

4. I will completely change my situation by driving my own car to work, dropping Jana off at preschool, and using that as my legitimate reason for ending my participation in the group commuter program.

Now you are ready to take a close, detailed look at the exact stimuli that contribute to your stress and the physical and emotional responses to each stimulus. On the blanks below write a brief description of each stimulus and each response.

STRESS STIMULI   PHYSICAL AND EMOTIONAL RESPONSES

1._____ _____

_____ _____

_____ _____

2._____ _____

_____ _____

_____ _____

3._____ _____

_____ _____

_____ _____

4._____ _____

_____ _____

_____ _____

Now you can begin the next step, which is writing *new* responses for each stress stimulus you have listed. Remember to *state your new response positively.* For example, let's suppose your stress stimulus is having to deal with your company president in a one-to-one situation, and your present responses are clammy hands, shaking voice, breathing difficulty, and feelings of inadequacy. Here is a negative new response for that stimulus:

When I am going to be in a one-to-one situation with the president, I will *try* to relax and I will *not* get nervous. I will *not* let him make me feel inadequate because I will hold my own.

Here is a positive new response for that same stimulus:

When I am going to be in a one-to-one situation with the president, I will breathe deeply and relax before entering his office. I will visualize myself as the successful and knowledgeable employee I am. I have a lot to contribute and I am relaxed as I make that contribution.

Now look back at your stress stimuli and responses and write your new responses, using the format shown in Chris's example. That is, your new response will start with an identification of the stimulus: "When my mother-in-law calls at breakfast, I will . . ." or "When my daughter acts as if she doesn't hear me, I will . . . " or "When my roommate plays the stereo at the same time I am studying, I will . . ."

Now write your new responses below, remembering to identify the stimulus as you begin your response.

NEW RESPONSES

1. _____

_____

_____

2. _____

_____

_____

3. _____

_____

_____

4. _____

_____

_____

Setting Up Your New Plan

Your overall objectives in regard to changing your behavior are clear. They are:

1. To reduce or eliminate negative stress in your life.
2. To incorporate new responses into your life.
3. To become a calmer, more effective, healthier person.

These are your general goals. To accomplish them, you need to reprogram your subconscious so it can help you act on and experience new responses to old stimuli. You need to:

Accept the repressed feelings that are causing you to feel anxious and irritable and to feel freedom as you accept those feelings. The induction suggests, "Let any feelings you have buried come up to the surface, and look at those feelings. See which ones you want to keep and which ones you don't want to keep. Keep the ones you need right now and cast away the others. It is all right for you to feel sad or depressed sometimes. It is a way of being good to yourself. The time will soon be over for those feelings and you will feel free from them. You can accept or discard any feelings at all, discard any feelings you are through with . . . "

Feel protected from outside pressures and stress. The induction suggests, "You are surrounded by a shield that protects you from pressure. The shield prevents outside pressure from invading you. Pressure bounces off, and away from you, bounces off and away. You feel fine because the shield protects you all day from stress and pressure."

Incorporate new responses into your life. The induction suggests, "You now have new responses to old situations." At this point in the induction, you will insert a stimulus and a new response for that stimulus. ("When [INSERT A STIMULUS] I will [INSERT NEW RESPONSE].") It is best to treat one stimulus at a time. You will see exactly where to place your new response in the induction which follows.

The Total Induction

Now that you understand how the induction works, you are ready to use it. The *Stress Reduction Induction* is used with the *Relaxation Induction* in Chapter 2. You may remember that the *Relaxation Induction* was divided into two parts. The *Stress Reduction Induction* comes *between* the two parts. The three components should not be separated from each other as they are used or taped; instead, they should blend into one another in a continuous flow. Keeping that in mind, follow this procedure:

1. Turn to Chapter 2. Use the *Going Down Induction*.

2. Use the *Stress Reduction Induction* that follows.

3. Turn to Chapter 2. Use the *Coming Up Induction.*

STRESS REDUCTION INDUCTION

Because you are now relaxed, let any feelings you have buried come up to the surface. Examine those feelings. Decide which ones you want to keep and which ones you want to discard. Keep the ones you need right now, and cast away the others. It is all right for you to feel sad or depressed sometimes. It is your way of being good to yourself. Depression is a healing process so you can allow yourself to mourn or be sad and when you have completed the time of sadness, set yourself free. You are good to yourself and the time will soon be over for those feelings and you will feel free from them. You will feel free because you can accept or discard any feelings at all, discard any feelings you are through with. They are yours, and you can let them come and go, come and go as you need them. Now relax, and continue to relax, and feel yourself relaxed with your feelings. And think of how you are a whole person with many feelings that make you whole and healthy. And if any unwanted outside pressure comes at you, you are surrounded by a shield that protects you from pressure. The shield will protect you from the pressure. The shield prevents outside pressure from invading you. Pressure bounces off and away from you, bounces off and away. No matter where it comes from or who sends it, it just bounces off and away. It bounces off and away. You feel fine because the shield protects you all day from stress and pressure. You go through your day feeling fine. You watch the stress bounce off and away. The more stress outside, the calmer you feel inside. The calmer you feel inside. Calm inside. You are a calm person and you are shielded from stress. You act in ways that make you feel good. You now have new responses to old situations. [INSERT ONE STIMULUS AND NEW RESPONSE.] *This new response will make you feel strong and calm and free. Your days will be full of accomplishments and you will be pleased with those accomplishments. You will feel good about yourself because you have new responses that are making your day more pleasant, you are calm and strong and free from stress. You are completely free from stress. You are free from stress.*

What to Expect and Following Up

Each time you have successfully reprogrammed a new response to an old stimulus, you can proceed to the next one on your list. A few sessions for each stimulus will no doubt be necessary. Except for the insertion of a new response, your *Stress Reduction Induction* will remain the same, reinforcing a feeling of protection from stress, affirming that you are a calmer, healthier person who is not afraid to feel necessary emotions.

After you have reprogrammed all of your new responses, the *Stress Reduction Induction* can be capsulized to suit your own needs. You may extract a part that is particularly suitable for you to use as stress maintenance; that is, a sort of mini-induction to serve as reinforcement during a particularly trying time. If you need to use the induction during an excessively stressful day, you can think your way through it, as explained in Chapter 2.

Generally, whenever you feel stress begin to build again, you should use the entire *Stress Reduction Induction*. If you recognize that your old patterns of behavior are creeping back into your life, then resume the induction until you no longer need it.

Laughter Therapy

In places of extreme stress—hospitals, war zones, sites of disaster— spontaneous humor is often evident. It is a way that people in intolerable situations deal with their stress, loss, and anxiety. Even though the humor is often grim, it works. It meets an immediate mental and emotional need and, in addition, is beneficial to the physical body. It relaxes the facial muscles and lungs and releases endorphins, the agents that increase a feeling of well-being.

In hypnotherapy work at a veteran's hospital, the patients were being treated and prepared for re-entry into the community. The *Stress Reduction* and *Relaxation Inductions* were producing a steady but slow modification in the veterans' behavior. When laughter therapy was added to stress reduction therapy, it made a strong, positive difference in behavior.

The hypnotherapist first asked the group members to think of a funny situation, a joke, or a comical movie. During the induction, some of the patients began to laugh aloud, the laughter quickly became contagious, and all the members of the group joined in. All the patients were animated and smiling. Even patients who had previously been extremely depressed joined in the laughter. Perhaps most important is the fact that this momentary improvement led to accelerated rehabilitation, resulting in permanent positive changes for most patients.

To incorporate humor into your induction, you may use an amusing incident from your past, an imaginary comical situation, jokes, a comedian's taped routine—anything you think is funny. You may begin the laughter therapy by using a suggestion similar to the following:

Recall a funny incident, a comedy movie, a joke you heard. Think about it and let yourself laugh, feeling the corners of your mouth turn up, letting yourself laugh, feeling laughter coming from your throat and rolling into a hearty laugh. Feel it vibrate through your body. When you finish laughing, experience a sense of release and well-being and keep that feeling of well-being with you throughout the day.

In addition to using laughter therapy within the *Stress Reduction Induction,* you may use it as a mini-induction whenever you feel the need for relief in an otherwise sober and intense day.

Case Study

Adrienne, a 55-year-old school administrator, was in the process of getting divorced when she was also put in the role of caring for her aging father, who was irritable and often downright illogical. The two were sharing Adrienne's house, and she had hired a housekeeper/companion to stay with her father during the day. When Adrienne returned home, she had usually experienced a day of demands, decision-making, and problem management. Her public relations skills had been fully operative from 7:45 A.M., when she entered her office, to 5:00 P.M. or later, when her day ended. Upon her arrival at home, her father's demands would begin. What in the world would they have for dinner, and where were the slacks Adrienne was supposed to pick up at the cleaners, and when would she have time to attend to her father's errands? When Adrienne went out once or twice a week, she was made to feel guilty for leaving her 80-year-old parent home alone.

Adrienne's life was made up of job requirements, stress, and guilt. As a result, she had high blood pressure and was generally unhappy. She sought relief in hypnotherapy. She had one session a week for four months. During the *Stress Reduction Induction* she was reprogrammed to imagine that she was encased in an armor that pressures could not penetrate. She also learned to visualize the comical side of irrational situations that had once caused great stress.

At the end of four months, she was much happier, affable, and able to see herself not as a victim but as a person with renewed power.

Special Considerations

Severe stress and depression are candidates for counseling as well as hypnotherapy, especially if the symptoms continue for a lengthy period of time. It should also be noted that the symptoms cited under the discussion of the PMS syndrome could be indicators of other physical problems as well. The safe approach is to check into any such symptoms to eliminate the possibility of a disorder that requires immediate medical treatment.

Finally, it is wise to remember that if your emotions are not given relief from stress, your body will soon feel the results.

7

Treating Phobias

One afternoon, Julie, a 34-year-old housewife, became extremely fearful and disoriented while shopping in a large department store. Julie's heart began to beat erratically. Breathing was difficult. She left the store quickly and went home to call her doctor. But once she had entered her house, her symptoms began to subside. Julie was experiencing the onset of *agoraphobia,* an abnormal fear of being in open places.

The same fear reoccurred the next week when Julie went to the supermarket. A few evenings later she attempted to go to a movie with her husband, but she panicked in the parking lot and they had to return home. Within a month Julie was afraid to venture outside her home. She had to develop a support system that would permit her to remain inside permanently. Her husband and neighbors ran all errands and did the necessary shopping. She stayed inside her home for twelve years before seeking professional help.

Julie's phobia is just one example of hundreds of obsessive and irrational fears of people, places, objects, or situations. The physical reactions vary in severity from mild to intense. Among the symptoms are sweaty palms, erratic heartbeat, nausea, increased muscle tension, shortness of breath, blurred vision, and fainting.

Distinguishing Harmless Fears From Phobias

Not all fears are harmful. In fact, many are even useful. For example, a four-year-old who has not been conditioned to fear traffic may stroll in front of a two-ton truck with the same ease with which he crosses the path of the family cat. In this case, fear is useful and beneficial for personal safety.

If a fear is useless, that does not necessarily indicate that it is harmful, either. In fact, there are useless fears that nearly all people seem to manifest from birth, such as the fear of snakes, spiders, and excessive heights. A person with a useless fear that is magnified into a single simple phobia can most often function quite well by avoiding the one object, animal, or situation that stimulates the fear. It is easy, for example, for a person to live with *pteronophobia, aulophobia,* or *batrachophobia.* One simply stays away from feathers, flutes, and frogs! If the phobia does not interfere with a person's emotional, social, or work life, then it may not require treatment.

To gauge the degree to which your fear is affecting you, ask yourself the following:

1. Is my fear taking up a lot of my time? Do I think about it obsessively?
2. Is my fear forcing me to do things the hard way? Do I drive to work using a route that takes me five miles out of my way, rather than panic in the Lincoln Tunnel?
3. Is my fear affecting the other relationships in my life? Do I avoid going to bed at the same time as my wife because I am extremely afraid of being impotent?
4. Is my fear affecting my physical condition? Do my hands shake frequently? Is my pulse often rapid? Do I get lots of headaches? Do I have blurred vision or nausea? Do I stutter? Am I often depressed?

If you responded yes to any of these questions, you are a likely candidate for treatment.

Unlocking the Phobia

A phobia may have established such a firm hold on your life that it seems impossible to unlock, or even understand. However, regardless of the specific stimulus that produces the fear—whether it be dogs, thunderstorms, cancer, the naked body, fire, death, or being touched by another person—the majority of phobias are generated from one of the following five causes:

Your phobia may be the product of severe stress. Stress can be repressed for such a long time or to such a degree that it surfaces in another form, that of irrational fear. You may be experiencing a great amount of stress in relation to a specific thing, place, or situation, but that stress may materialize as a phobia about some *other* thing, place, or situation. For example, Brent developed a fear of crossing a particular bridge in town. As a junior attorney in a large law firm, Brent experienced a great degree of "invisible" pressure at work, and often felt victimized in personal confrontations with the firm's senior partners. The office of the law firm was located across the dreaded bridge. By developing an abnormal fear of the bridge, Brent avoided acknowledging the real cause of severe stress, his job.

Helen, a research analyst in her forties, was extremely shy and had difficulty relating to people. After several social encounters that she perceived as torturous, she developed a fear of driving at night. This fear allowed her to escape from most forms of social activity. Both Brent and Helen transferred stress from one area of life to another, which resulted in what could be called "displaced" phobias. Often in this type of stress-based fear the person selects something that can be easily avoided as the object of the phobia, rather than fearing a true stimulus that is difficult or impossible to avoid. Thus a nine-year-old girl may fear bicycling, which can be avoided, when the true object of her fear is her grandfather, who cannot be avoided.

Your phobia may be the product of a series of experiences occurring over a period of years, which have built up into an excessive anxiety. Many fears related to your own performance or to being in certain social situations can cause you to build up a fear of phobic proportions. You may think of this cause as an accumulation of distressing events that perpetuate and increase a state of dread.

Carl's worst fear involved playing sports. When he was eight years old and tried to skate, he immediately fell, skinning his face. When Carl was ten, an older boy taunted him throughout a neighborhood baseball game. When he was a freshman in high school, the track coach told him he needed to build up his muscles. He was instructed to run laps while the other members of the team were competing with one another in a trial meet. By the time Carl was a sophomore, he was terrified of failure, dreaded physical education of any sort, and became nauseated when he had to perform in front of others.

This type of personal history, which includes a series of negative experiences that reinforce each other, can culminate in a phobia that may transfer or radiate to other areas of life.

Your phobia may be the product of a fear of fear. "We have nothing to fear but fear itself" is more than a piece of rhetoric. If you have a fear of panic, of fear itself, it is a very real phobia. Your fear can be associated with anything and everything because you believe that as you go over a certain threshold of stress in the presence of a certain stimulus, you will panic. By anticipating panic, you raise your stress level and the fear of fear turns into a destructive cycle. You avoid so many situations in your effort not to be afraid that your life becomes very limited. You may be afraid to go downtown, afraid to talk to certain people, afraid to have a job, afraid of traveling, afraid of parenting. Nothing is exempt from your fear, and your activities become increasingly restricted as the fear radiates into all facets of your life.

Your phobia may have been transmitted to you by another person. This cause of phobias is probably the easiest to understand, because it is imposed on you by an outside force. For example, if you continually see your father react with horror to thunderstorms, you are likely to react the same way. In this case, you have "caught" the fear from someone who serves as a role model for you.

Anyone with whom you are in close contact—a friend, neighbor, or even a stranger—can transmit a fear. If you observe that the man in your apartment building always panics at the sight of the elevator and must use the stairs, you may eventually begin to fear elevators yourself.

Your phobia may be the result of a severe past trauma. A painful emotional experience from the past can produce an unreasonable fear of that same situation, object, person, or place that originally caused the fear. The trauma can be either conscious or subconscious; that is, you may be aware of the original cause of the fear, or you may have successfully buried the trauma and have no conscious recollection of it. In many cases, the trauma that caused the phobia is repressed.

Paul, a 62-year-old sales representative for an electronics firm, suffered from *claustrophobia,* a common but abnormal fear of enclosed or narrow places. For thirty years he had been afraid of being inside elevators, trains, airplanes, and cars or of having to climb enclosed staircases. He was unable to take a shower unless someone else was present in the same room. Using the *Age Regression Induction,* which is included in this chapter, he recalled an incident from his childhood when a babysitter punished him by locking him in his bedroom closet. In the dark, he imagined that he shared the closet with evil monsters who were whispering, planning their vicious attack on him. As an adult, Paul carried that original fear whenever he was spatially confined in any way.

Ann, a 39-year-old graphic illustrator, had a phobia regarding relationships with men. The mere thought of making a commitment to a man gave her anxiety attacks. To avoid a positive relationship that might require a commitment (or at least offer the chance for the pursuit of some degree of pleasure), Ann chose men who were abusive. If she happened to be involved with a sensitive and caring man, she would feel unworthy of his affection, begin fearing that he would leave her, and terminate the relationship.

During the *Age Regression Induction,* Ann recalled memories that had been repressed for 33 years. Her father had beaten and molested her when she was between the ages of four and six. Ann's mother had left her spouse soon after, but her daughter had already been damaged in several ways. She had developed a distorted view of what a successful relationship should be, as she had come to think that if she directed all of her efforts toward pleasing her father she could win his approval and he would stop his assaults. As an adult, Ann continued to try to gain approval from men whose character closely resembled that of her father. During hypnotherapy, Ann was helped by visualizing past events and severing her emotional ties with them.

In cases of molestation, rape, and child abuse, hypnotic age regression has tremendous value because it motivates recall of repressed memories and traumas, which are then exposed and can be dealt with. Once the scenes and situations are made available, the phobic can sever emotional ties with them.

All past traumas, however, do not emerge from childhood. You may have a past trauma that has developed as a result of your divorce seven years ago, the birth of your first child last year, your mother's death a decade ago, or your move to a different city last Christmas. The common characteristic for all traumas is the same. It is an event, incident, or period of time that cannot be consciously recalled without provoking alarm, extreme anxiety, or panic.

Getting Rid of Your Phobia

Regardless of your type of phobia, there are several major steps that you can take to rid yourself of the fear.

You may want to identify the specific event that caused the fear and sever your emotional ties to it. This procedure, which is called age regression, is not recommended for everyone. It is presented here as an *option.* If your fear originated from an extremely traumatic situation, it may be to your advantage to leave it alone. Examining its origin may bring other emotional problems to the surface.

A procedure for testing the personal value and safety of using the *Age Regression Induction* is explained in the material that follows. If you decide to go ahead with this technique, remember that there is no need to try to force a memory, or focus on a specific age as you search for clues to your fear. As you use the *Age Regression Induction,* the incident will surface on its own, and it will be recognizable as the original cause. The induction suggests, "Let your mind drift back in time. See yourself at the age you were when you first experienced your fear. Ask yourself, 'Is this the first time I felt my fear?' If the answer is no, go back until it feels as if you are recalling the right incident. Place it on a movie screen in front of you. Imagine yourself connected to that screen by a cord. Now cut the cord."

Notice that in using this technique you may need to scan backwards, stopping several times along the way to question yourself about whether or not the experience you are recalling constitutes the true origin of your phobia.

The case of John, "The Spider Man," serves as an excellent example of how the *Age Regression Induction* works. John is a 36-year-old successful businessman who is married and has two children. He suffered from a fear of spiders most of his life. When he was under stress, the fear intensified into a kind of panic. He had nightmares about spiders attacking him, and he was in a constant state of anxiety, fearing that a spider might crawl on him before he could be alerted to its prescence. The phobia was disrupting his normal routine to such a degree that he decided to visit a hypnotherapist.

John believed the cause of his fear was an incident in his childhood when a neighbor frightened the young children in the neighborhood by chasing them with rubber spiders. However, John was anxious to investigate the exact origin of the trauma while he was in a hypnotic state. In the first few sessions, the *Relaxation Induction* was used. As John's stress was reduced through relaxation, his nightmares lessened. In the next few sessions, the *Age Regression Induction* was introduced, and John scanned his childhood.

John's first spider-related memory was of the neighbor chasing the small children across his lawn, while holding a large rubber spider. At this point the question was put to John, "Is this the first time you felt the fear of spiders?" Without disturbing his trance state, John answered no.

He continued to regress to earlier ages, and each memory described an event that frightened him. In one memory, John had gone down the stairs of his basement at home. He found an old box that contained his father's Army paraphernalia, including medals, an old uniform, and a hat. While he was searching through these items, a spider jumped out of the uniform and crawled over John's hand. Again, he was asked the question, "Is this the first time your were frightened by a spider?" Again John answered no. The regression continued until John remembered his earliest incident. He was five years old, playing in a deserted train yard. As he crawled over some rubble, a large dark hand, its fingers resembling the legs of a huge spider, reached out from the debris and grabbed him around the leg. John fought and struggled until he pulled free, and then ran home. He was not supposed to have been playing in the train yard, so he didn't tell his parents about the episode. John successfully put the traumatic incident out of his conscious mind.

Once John realized what had happened to cause his phobia, the next step was for him to let go of the old emotional tie to that memory. To accomplish this, John viewed the event on a movie screen in his imagination. He visualized being connected to the screen by a cord, which he then cut loose.

Confront your fear while experiencing it as a nonthreatening experience. The *Confrontation Induction,* which follows, suggests, "Imagine yourself face to face with your fear. You are at ease. You are smiling because your fear has lost its strength, its importance, you no longer need it and you no longer want it."

Increase your self-confidence. Confidence goes hand in hand with not experiencing an abnormal degree of fear. The *Confrontation Induction* also suggests, "You are confident, you can face anything, and you have tremendous inner strength. All you need to do whenever you feel anxious is to feel a powerful surge of strength within."

Reprogram your subconscious, using a positive posthypnotic suggestion in regard to your specific fear. The imagery you use for your suggestion will depend, of course, on your phobia. Your individualized posthypnotic suggestion will describe the situation that causes the fear, but each part of the situation will be pleasant, and your reaction to it will be positive.

Treating Your Specific Phobia, a later section in this chapter, includes posthypnotic suggestions to use within your major induction.

In several of the posthypnotic suggestions (for the fear of crossing bridges, driving, enclosed spaces, and so on), you use a technique called *pair bonding,* in which you pair up a past positive experience with the present negative experience that causes your abnormal fear. You then permit the negative stimulus (the bridge, the elevator) to serve as a cue to all the pleasant emotions that went with the past positive experience. By linking the two experiences together, the positive one serves to counteract your fear and eventually modify your reaction to the phobia stimulus.

How you use the posthypnotic suggestions will be explained in detail in the material which follows. If your specific fear is not included, you can create your own posthypnotic suggestion by using those in the section as models and reviewing the *Guidelines for Effective Suggestions* in Chapter 3.

Your Plan of Attack

Because phobias can be developed in response to any imaginable situation, or any person, place, or thing in our world, it would be impossible to present *one* induction which would be effective for all phobias. Therefore, the major induction that you will use to treat your specific fear will be made up of either four or five components. It will consist of four components if the cause of your phobia is known, and five components if the origin is the result of a repressed past trauma.

As you record your induction, follow these steps:

1. Turn to Chapter 2 and use the *Going Down Induction*.

2. If you are not consciously aware of an origin for your fear, you may wish to use the *Age Regression Induction* in this chapter.

3. Use the *Confrontation Induction* in this chapter.

4. Look at the section, *Treating Your Specific Phobia,* in this chapter. Find a description of the specific fear that you want to eliminate. Review the specific objectives you need to achieve and read the posthypnotic suggestion for your fear. Following the guidelines below, personalize your posthypnotic suggestion and record it after the *Confrontation Induction.* As you record the suggestion, you should repeat the key phrases within the suggestion and then repeat the whole suggestion a second time.

5. Close with the *Coming Up Induction* from Chapter 2.

These components should be recorded so they flow together to make the whole. They will work together to meet your individual needs. Item 1 provides relaxation. Item 2 helps locate the origin of the fear, which has been hidden in your subconscious. Item 3 helps you meet your fear face to face in a positive situation and to gain power over it. Item 4 addresses your specific problem in detail and reprograms your subconscious so that you may experience a permanent change in your behavior. Item 5 brings you out of the induction in a relaxed and pleasant state.

The suggestions in the *Treating Your Specific Phobia* section are presented there as models. You should expand upon the theme of the suggestion you select; that is, it can serve as a core, around which you build a thoroughly effective posthypnotic induction. What you insert into this suggestion or add on to it is determined by the particular circumstances that surround your specific fear As you develop a personalized posthypnotic suggestion, remember to employ the key components of an induction, as explained in Chapter 2. Use *synonyms* for reinforcement, *paraphrase your suggestions, use connective words* to maintain a steady flow of language, and *designate time* ("in just a few moments," "now you will . . .") when you need to signal the beginning or end of a particular behavior. (Note: If your fear is not included in this section, find a fear similar to yours and read the posthypnotic suggestion for that fear. Then, using it as a model, write your own suggestion by referring to *Guidelines for Effective Suggestions* in Chapter 3.)

Using the Age Regression Induction

A phobia may have a deep emotional origin, and treating it may bring other emotional problems to the surface. For this reason, the guidance of a psychologist can be extremely beneficial. Counseling will help you determine the appropriate procedures for treatment.

If you decide to investigate your subconscious to excavate the trauma or traumas that first caused your phobia, you need to ask your subconscious if it is permissible for you to find the cause of your phobia and if it will be a beneficial experience for you. You need to find out if it is *valuable* and *safe*. If the answer is yes, then you can proceed; if the answer is no, if you feel that delving into your past may be harmful, then you need to reconsider the course of your action.

To communicate with your subconscious, you will use "ideomotor finger signals." First, make yourself comfortable and relaxed by using the *Relaxation Induction* from Chapter 2. When you have become completely relaxed, focus your attention on your fingers. Repeat the word yes . . . yes . . . yes, over and over and notice which finger is your "yes" finger. Keep thinking the word yes, and soon you will notice a little tug or twitch or sensation in one of your ten fingers—that will be your "yes" finger. Now repeat the word "no" over and over, while watching for any sensation, twitch, or movement in another finger. That will be your "no" finger.

At this point you can ask your subconscious for permission to seek information regarding your phobia. Ask your subconscious if it is beneficial for you to regress in order to discover the origin of your phobia. If you feel movement or sensation in your "yes" finger, you can proceed by allowing your mind to drift back to the very first time you experienced your fear. If your subconscious gives you a "no" signal, leave the source of your phobia alone and continue to deal only with the phobia itself, using the other methods in this chapter.

AGE REGRESSION INDUCTION

Let your mind drift back in time, and as you begin to drift easily, easily back in time, see yourself become younger and younger, and know that you are safe. You are protected by your own positive energy, you may view past experiences as if you are a spectator, you may view past experiences from a safe distance, you need only remember that you are in control, you can see past fears at a distance, you can see them up close or you don't have to see them at all, if you choose to terminate your session, all you need to do is count from one to ten and return to full consciousness. However, if you are ready to proceed, just let your mind drift back and think about your fear, your phobia, what frightens you, and know that here and now you are safe, you view yourself as a detective, you are curious, eager to learn of the origin of your fear, eager to investigate all clues. Go back in time, go back to the first time you experienced your fear, see it at a distance, you might imagine seeing it on a movie screen at a safe distance, you are feeling fine, you begin to understand why you felt fearful, small pieces of the puzzle begin to fit. As you view the first episode of your fear, ask your fingers, "Is this the very first time I felt my fear?" [PAUSE.] *If your finger says no, continue to go back further into time, see yourself become younger and younger and go back to the next incident that caused you to become fearful, again see it on a screen at a distance. You are safe, you are a spectator viewing your past. You gain more understanding with each recall. Again, ask your fingers the question, "Is this the first time I felt my fear?"* [PAUSE.] *If the answer is no, go back until you recall the incident that caused your phobia. When you have reached a time that feels as if it might be the one you are searching for, ask your subconscious, "Is this the first time I felt my fear?"* [PAUSE.] *If your finger says yes, view the incident on the screen at a distance, when you begin to feel more comfortable and know the past has no influence on you in the present, view the incident and begin to understand why you became fearful. As you learn about your past, let the screen come a little closer to you, at a comfortable distance from you, and now begin to let go and release old emotional ties to the past, let go of fear, let go of anger, let go of pain, as you release old emotional ties to the past, you allow the screen to come closer and closer, and the memories are losing their hold on you and whenever you are ready you can imagine a cord connected from you to the screen, a cord that ties you to the past, now just imagine cutting the cord, cutting the cord to the screen, you are cutting the cord to the screen and releasing yourself from the past, just watch the screen fade away, the screen grows more and more faint, the screen is dim and disappearing and as the screen fades you begin to feel a healing take place, healing from past fears and past experiences, healing and soothing, and now your body, your mind, your heart, your whole self is free of your old fear. You are completely free, you no longer need your fear, your fear has disappeared, disappeared, your phobia has lost its strength and it is deflated like an empty balloon, and now you are totally and completely free and you feel relieved as if a burden has been lifted from your shoulders, you feel at ease, completely free, your old fear is gone, gone, completely free, and now you are completely free and now you are completely free and you will continue to experience this freedom.*

CONFRONTATION INDUCTION

Imagine yourself face-to-face with your fear. Make your fear into something you can see. Now look at it and notice how weak it is, it is very weak, very weak. You are much stronger than it is, much stronger. In fact, it is afraid of you because you are much stronger than it is, much stronger. You are at ease, completely at ease, and strong. You are smiling because your fear has lost its strength, its importance, you no longer need it and you no longer want it. You do not want it. Imagine your life without it. You live happily, you are confident, very confident because you can face anything and you know you have tremendous inner strength. All you need to do whenever you feel anxious is to breathe deeply, relax, and feel a powerful surge of strength within. You smile and your stress melts away. You are capable and confident and in charge.

TREATING YOUR SPECIFIC PHOBIA

Follow the guidelines provided in the *Your Plan of Attack* section to personalize and record the specific posthypnotic suggestion for your phobia.

FEAR OF CROWDS

[OBJECTIVE: To foster a sense of well-being; to relieve anxiety about groups of people; to regard other people as nonthreatening.]

Imagine yourself safe within a crowd. You can mingle easily, you enjoy the crowd, and you know that you can extract yourself any time you please. You feel free and comfortable being close to people.

FEAR OF AN ANIMAL

[OBJECTIVE: To view a specific animal as nonthreatening; to appreciate its appearance and qualities; to appreciate it for what it is.]

You are near a [NAME ANIMAL]. *You look into the animal's eyes, and you are calm and relaxed. You admire the animal's fur, its body structure, the way it moves, the noises it makes. You reach out and touch it; it is calm. This* [NAME ANIMAL] *seems to like being in your presence. You reach out and touch it and it is calm, very calm.*

FEAR OF THE OPPOSITE SEX

[OBJECTIVE: To build self-esteem and foster a feeling of personal security; to view interaction with the opposite sex as a positive experience.]

Imagine that another person has all the positive characteristics you could want in a partner. You and the other person have similar interests and desires and are responsive to each other. Both of you can communicate your feelings and desires and you are responsive to each other. Both of you can communicate very well. You are open to intimacy. You are now ready to have a loving and fulfilling relationship. You reject all that is harmful or negative because from now on you are open only to positive feelings.

FEAR OF DARKNESS

[OBJECTIVE: To remove the anxiety regarding the unknown or mysterious quality of darkness; to encourage perception of darkness as a comfort and a necessity.]

The dark places around you are the same places that you can see in the daytime. These places are just put into shadow, put into rest for awhile. Darkness is a comfortable blanket that falls over everything. Darkness helps us relax. It is a pleasant change from the full light of day. We need the darkness because it helps us rest and sleep.

FEAR OF CROSSING BRIDGES

[OBJECTIVE: To associate a feared experience with a positive experience from the past; to instill a feeling of control and strength.]

Reflect on your past successes and your capability. Think about your strength. You can do anything that you want to do. Recall a time and place that was soothing and calm. This same calm feeling will return when you are approaching a bridge and it will stay with you all the way across the bridge. Now imagine yourself crossing that bridge from one side to the other with that same calm, soothing feeling you had when you [INSERT THE CALM EXPERIENCE FROM THE PAST].

FEAR OF DRIVING

[USE THE *Crossing Bridges* SUGGESTION, SUBSTITUTING A DRIVING EXPERIENCE.]

FEAR OF HEIGHTS

[USE THE *Crossing Bridges* SUGGESTION, SUBSTITUTING AN EXPERIENCE THAT INVOLVES HEIGHT.]

FEAR OF ENCLOSED SPACES

[OBJECTIVE: To associate a feared experience with a positive experience from the past; to instill a feeling of control and strength.]

You are in a car, feeling calm, feeling relaxed and enjoying where you are, and looking forward to traveling. You are in a small room and you feel strong, the same way you felt when you were [INSERT THE POSITIVE EXPERIENCE FROM THE PAST].

FEAR OF OPEN SPACES

[OBJECTIVE: To associate a feared experience with a positive experience from the past; to foster enjoyment of open spaces.]

You are in a park, feeling relaxed, standing in the open, enjoying the fresh air, the sunshine, the space around you. You feel just as calm as you did when you [INSERT THE POSITIVE EXPERIENCE FROM THE PAST]. *It feels good to be out in the open. You can take a walk or jog, or just sit and enjoy the peacefulness of your surroundings. You are relaxed and in control and enjoying yourself.*

FEAR OF WATER

[OBJECTIVE: To associate a feared experience with a positive experience from the past; to instill a feeling of control and strength; to foster enjoyment of being in water.]

See yourself entering the water of a lake. You are smiling and confident and you are there to enjoy yourself. You need only go in as far as you like, and you always have the option to come out. You feel just as calm and relaxed as you did when you [INSERT THE POSITIVE EXPERIENCE FROM THE PAST]. *You enjoy yourself, the water is relaxing. You are safe, confident, and strong.*

FEAR OF INCONTINENCE

[OBJECTIVE: To instill confidence about having control over bodily processes.]

ımagine your bowel becoming stronger and stronger and you are gaining control over all of your bodily organs. They function with your permission and your permission only. You are fine, your body is completely under your control.

FEAR OF BEING ALONE

[OBJECTIVE: To increase self-reliance; to make solitude appealing, enjoyable, and safe.]

You are a capable person who can deal with any situation very effectively. You enjoy being alone because then you can do anything you please. You can do all the things you enjoy the most. The quiet and solitude are peaceful, restful, relaxing, and you feel relaxed and strong and happy by yourself. In this quiet place, alone, you allow yourself to think about your plans, dreams, and accomplishments.You allow yourself to do anything you like. You are completely at peace.

FEAR OF BEING TOUCHED

[OBJECTIVE: To relieve anxiety about intimacy; to foster acceptance of affection and appropriate physical contact.]

You are a warm, likable person who feels comfortable with other people, who likes being included in activities, who enjoys hugging a close friend. You enjoy hugging someone you care for, and you enjoy it when that person hugs you or touches you. When you are touched you feel a pleasant connection with your friends and those you love.

FEAR OF CHILDBIRTH

[SEE Chapter 8.]

FEAR OF DISEASE

[OBJECTIVE: To program a feeling of well-being and wholeness; to instill belief in having protection against illness and disease.]

Your body is healthy and strong, free of any trace of illness. You look in the mirror and your complexion is good. Your eyes are clear and sparkling. You look vital and wholesome. You feel energetic and you have lots of stamina. Your body feels great.

FEAR OF HEART ATTACKS

[OBJECTIVE: To promote a feeling of physical well-being; to encourage an average amount of physical exertion; to perceive the heart's condition as healthy and normal.]

Your whole body feels strong and energetic. You have lots of stamina and you feel the power available in your own body. You enjoy the exercise that is part of your daily routine, such as walking and climbing stairs. You can take long walks now and climb stairs now and you can do it with ease because you have a strong, healthy body. Your heart is strong and sure, its beat is as regular as the ticking of a clock. You will live a long and healthy life and you will enjoy many physical activities, you will enjoy any activities you choose.

FEAR OF BEING POISONED

[OBJECTIVE: To regard eating as a positive activity; to see foods as safe, desirable, delicious, and nourishing; to promote the enjoyment of dining out.]

You enter a restaurant and you like the way it looks. The aromas from the kitchen are tantalizing. They make you hungry. You are shown to a beautiful table overlooking a garden. You look at the menu and everything sounds delicious. You order and when your plate arrives your food is healthful, attractive, and appetizing. You can enjoy a leisurely, delicious meal, eating slowly and relishing the appealing flavors.

FEAR OF FEAR

[OBJECTIVE: To instill a feeling of well-being; to establish an emergency procedure for use in threatening situations; to promote an immunity to abnormal fear and vulnerability.]

Imagine yourself being in control of all situations, being in control of all the parts of your daily routine. If you ever feel that you are losing control you always have the tools to regain it. You stop, breathe deeply, relax, and you feel that shield around you, the shield that protects you from fear. No fear can get through that shield. The fear just melts away when it reaches the shield, the fear just dissolves and flows away.

What to Expect and Following Up

You may begin by using your induction once a day for several weeks, then less frequently as your fear begins to subside. You may need only one or two sessions to be free of your fear and never experience it again. Conversely, if no immediate change occurs, you may need to use the induction for several months.

After your fear has disappeared, periodically review your state of mind so that you may avoid any reoccurrence of the phobia or the manifestation of a new one. Check in with yourself on a regular basis to see if you are under stress. If you are, do something about it. Change your activity, allow yourself some kind of reward, relax, take a short vacation—or even a long one! If your stress is strong enough to be interfering with your life and causing emotional or physical problems, use the *Stress Reduction Induction* in Chapter 6.

Special Considerations

When treating your phobia, become aware of the other aspects of your life. Consider the foods you eat. Many foods can cause mood swings, depression, paranoia, anger, or fear. Foods that are high in glucose and foods that contain certain dyes are known to contribute to erratic behavior. Hormone imbalances can cause phobic reactions. In some cases a phobia may be a cover-up for an extremely deep-seated problem that needs extensive psychotherapy. Explore your entire health and use hypnotherapy as an independent tool or as an aid to accompany other types of mental and emotional care.

If you are treating others, don't force the phobic to consciously experience the fear-producing situation or confront the object of the phobia. While confrontation in a positive, pleasant, subconscious condition can be beneficial, actually living through the fear may serve to reinforce it. Don't express amusement, shock, or disbelief in regard to a phobic's specific fear stimulus. Remember, it can be anything from the color blue to an obscure venereal disease. Invoking shame, ridicule, or humor will inhibit or even terminate any progress. Throughout the period of treatment, it is important to emphasize that a person who can control and eliminate a fear is one who will experience benefits as he or she copes with other aspects of life that require persistence and strength.

8

Natural Childbirth

You are going to be asked to participate in a quick word association game. Look at the word below and say aloud the first word that pops into your mind:

labor

Now do the same for:

hospital

Common associations for the above are *labor–hard, hospital–sick.* (Your responses were probably similar, if not identical.)

These two associations are ones that natural childbirth successfully contradicts. Labor does not have to be a difficult, hard task. A mother-to-be is usually in the *hospital,* but she is not *sick* and should not be treated as if she were. Natural childbirth training encourages the mother to regard labor and delivery as a time of activity, concentration, and confidence, rather than a time of passivity and suffering. Anesthetics are kept to a minimum or are completely absent. Without drugs, the woman can assume an active role in the birth process. She can experience childbirth as a fulfilling and positive event.

When hypnosis is linked with natural childbirth training, double benefits result. These two methods of preparation do the following:

- Reduce or eliminate fear
- Produce pervasive relaxation
- Significantly diminish the need for medication; make possible complete elimination of medication for some subjects
- Make possible the complete control of uterine contractions
- Shorten the period of labor
- Lessen the behavioral signs of pain
- Promote a speedy recovery
- Foster and increase positive emotions during the entire birth process
- Create an experience which has highly charged spiritual or mystical qualities
- Stimulate and maintain a strong energy level into the post-delivery phase

It is important to understand that hypnosis works *with* natural childbirth techniques. It is most effective in partnership with the Lamaze or Bradley method. (If you are not already familiar with the specifics of natural childbirth, you will find an abundance of related reading material in bookstores and libraries.) Briefly, the natural methods allow you to develop effective breathing and relaxation techniques. The exercises suggested in any natural childbirth program should be followed on a regular basis, as recommended. They are designed specifically to help you build up muscle support during pregnancy, contribute to effective pushing during labor, and provide healthy muscle tone after birth. One of the major results of controlling the muscles during labor is a more regulated, comfortable birth. The breathing techniques you learn prior to childbirth teach you to respond to uterine contractions with controlled, relaxed breathing. This helpful activity takes your mind away from the discomfort of contractions and maintains a balanced amount of oxygen and carbon dioxide in your system. Through breathing and muscle control, you *coregulate* the birth process, rather than submit to being regulated by it.

The hypnosis–natural childbirth partnership can produce maximum results if you take the care, time and energy to create the necessary support system for this partnership. You need to:

Maintain good nutrition. It is easy to forget during pregnancy that the food you ingest contains the only nutrients your baby will receive. Your baby *becomes* what you eat.

In addition, good nutrition during pregnancy has other purposes besides supplying the necessary vitamins and minerals to the baby. It also:

- Provides strength, heat and energy for you
- Replaces worn out cells in your body
- Helps regulate your kidneys and bowels
- Maintains or improves the condition of your skin
- Prepares your system for nursing

Therefore, it is important for you to increase your protein intake and eat foods high in folic acid (raw, green, leafy vegetables). A lack of folic acid results in a type of anemia which is not corrected by an increase in iron.

You should also be especially aware of increasing your calcium (milk and yogurt) intake. As your baby's bones calcify in the last four and a half months of pregnancy, the need for calcium increases. If you do not ingest enough calcium to provide a supplemental supply to your baby, the calcium will come from your own bones and teeth. Some even claim that calcium has the added benefit of serving as a pain buffer. Old medical textbooks, for example, advised injections of calcium to serve as a pain killer for pleurisy.

Foods with plenty of iron (beef, liver, oysters, spinach) are important, but even if you eat these foods frequently you cannot assume that your iron intake is sufficient. It is wise to have your iron checked and to ask your doctor or other health professional to recommend an iron supplement as well as a prenatal vitamin.

Shield yourself from stress. Stress during pregnancy can affect you and your baby. It is associated with many complications during pregnancy, childbirth, and the postpartum period. It has also been proven that stress affects the immune system and reduces your natural defense against infection and disease.

The *Relaxation Induction* in Chapter 2 will keep you feeling balanced, at ease, and pleasantly in control. The relaxation that occurs during the induction can be as beneficial as one to two hours of sleep.

You may not be fortunate enough to escape a situation in which you are overworked, under pressure, or separated from people who could serve as a support system. If this is your case, severe stress may threaten your state of well-being, no matter how aware you are of avoiding it. Any specific stress stimuli can be dealt with using the procedures outlined in Chapter 6.

Rest and sleep. You may be more tired during the first few months of pregnancy than you are in the latter months. Because your body is undergoing radical changes, you should acknowledge your need for rest. Your ability to relax in general and relax on cue during labor will be aided by your afternoon naps and eight hours of sleep each night. If you go to the birth process with a rested body, you will have more strength and stamina, and you will have a greater ability to focus and manage your emotions.

Maintain a positive attitude. Your attitude plays a tremendous role in the ease or difficulty of your pregnancy, as well as the length and severity of your labor. You would be a very unusual pregnant woman if you did not experience some emotional changes or sudden mood swings. Don't blame yourself; instead, try to recognize that irritability, tenseness, and frequent tears are, for the most part, a product of hormonal changes. So, while keeping your feelings in perspective, acknowledge them. (Don't react as Woody Allen described in *Manhattan:* "I can't express anger. That's one of the problems I have. I grow a tumor instead.") Once your negative emotion is recognized, give it a little time to air itself, then combat it with a strong, positive thought. Think about an aspect of your life that is going well, one that is providing you with something you need—emotionally, socially, intellectually, or financially.

The Pain Factor

All the preceding actions and conditions contribute to the positive birthing experience. If these actions are realized and the conditions are met, hypnosis and childbirth will work in conjunction with each other to:

1. Allow you to experience a healthy, positive pregnancy
2. Reduce or eliminate pain
3. Provide the ingredients for a successful birth experience
4. Enjoy a rewarding, pleasant postbirth phase

Of the four goals, none is more important than the second. Because of the magnitude of this objective, it deserves especially close scrutiny.

Most people associate birth with pain. When a woman begins labor, this association leads her to respond to her sensations as she would to pain. However, the brain will register painful sensations when it receives only one strong stimulus at a time. This means that signals from several strong stimuli can act as distractors that alleviate or eliminate the sensation of pain. The following exercise demonstrates this point.

Pinch the fleshy part of your hand between your thumb and your forefinger. Pinch only hard enough to notice a slight painful sensation. Concentrate on the pain. Do not think of anything else, only the pain.

Now stop for a moment. Direct your attention to a picture on the wall. Look at the picture and, at the same time, pinch your hand again, exerting the same amount of pressure. Continue to pinch, concentrating solely on the picture. Study the picture's content, color, design, shape, and detail. As you concentrate on something other than your hand, you will notice that your hand seems less painful. You may not notice any uncomfortable sensation at all. Although birthing pains are certainly more severe than a pinch, hypnosis allows you to use the same "redirection technique" during delivery. You can train yourself to divert your attention and be successful in reducing or eliminating the painful sensation.

During labor, the uterus contracts. The message of this stimulus is sent to the brain, and the brain selects a response. The most basic response to pain is tension, which magnifies the unwanted sensation. The untrained woman has no other response to use. If she has not learned to divert her attention from the pain, she has nothing to concentrate on except the contractions.

But you have an alternative: You can reinterpret the pain. During labor, when the message of the contraction reaches the brain, your new response will be controlled relaxation and correct breathing, as learned in your natural childbirth training. You can use the added resources of the hypnotic relaxation training, and you can use the positive imagery which you will learn in the *Childbirth Induction* in this chapter. You can enter into the birthing process well-equipped for total success.

Programming for Results

The *Childbirth Induction* is designed to help you think, feel and act in certain ways. The induction programs your subconscious by offering suggestions. Below are the specific objectives you will accomplish.

You will relax. The first part of the induction provides physical and emotional relaxation, which releases normal stress and helps you to remain calm throughout your pregnancy, as well as after delivery. The induction suggests, "Make yourself comfortable and relax all of the muscles in your body, from the top of your head to the tips of your toes."

You may communicate with your unborn baby. Some people believe that a woman and her baby are not only physically connected, but emotionally and spiritually connected as well. If you accept this belief, then it is important to use those emotional and spiritual connections. You can do this by letting your baby know that it is loved and wanted. The induction suggests, "Think about how much you want your baby and how much love you have to give your baby. Now just imagine directing that love to your baby, surrounding the womb with love, imagine this love to be a soothing pastel light that envelopes your baby."

You will program your mind for pain control. As previously explained, you can disassociate yourself from pain by shifting your attention to anther place, one that is far away from the discomfort produced by the sensations of the contractions. The induction directs you to your special place, a place of peace and calm. It can be near the ocean, in a forest, a meadow, any location that produces feelings of peacefulness in you. It does not have to be a real place; it can be an imaginary environment you have created. (See *Guided Imagery Suggestions: A Supplement* in Chapter 3.) The induction suggests, "Whenever you feel discomfort, you take your thought far away to your special place, you breathe evenly, you know exactly what needs to be done. You feel yourself push and breathe and you feel comfortable, in charge."

You will experience a successful delivery. Chances of a speedier and easier delivery are increased with positive imagery. The induction suggests, "Your delivery is successful in every way, in every way, and when the baby arrives it is healthy and strong."

You will enjoy a positive postbirth phase. A loss of energy, a hormonal imbalance, a lack of confidence, a poor self-image, or even the normal demands of motherhood can be responsible for the postbirth blues. The last part of the induction is designed to help you maintain a positive feeling after childbirth and to strengthen your self-image. The induction suggests, "Imagine yourself home with your baby, you are a natural mother, you know instinctively how to care for your child. You accept the changes in your life with enthusiasm, you see difficulties as challenges. Just see yourself smiling, feeling good about yourself and your life, and see yourself as the attractive, capable, and loving woman whom you are."

The Total Induction

Now that you understand how the induction works, you are ready to use it. The *Childbirth Induction* is used with the *Relaxation Induction* in Chapter 2. You may remember that the *Relaxation Induction* was divided into two parts. The *Childbirth Induction* comes *between* the two parts. The three components should not be separated from one another as they are used or taped; instead, they should blend into one another in one continuous flow. Keeping that in mind, follow this procedure:

1. Turn to Chapter 2. Use the *Going Down Induction.*

2. Use the *Childbirth Induction* in this chapter.

3. Turn to Chapter 2. Use the *Coming Up Induction.*

CHILDBIRTH INDUCTION

Imagine your special place and feel a sense of peace and calm flow through you. You feel relaxed, your back feels relaxed, your stomach feels relaxed and your baby is calm and relaxed and now let yourself drift and float into a comfortable state of relaxation and bring to your mind the tremendous love you feel for your baby. [PAUSE.] *Just think about how much you want your baby and how much love you have to give your baby.* [PAUSE.] *Now just imagine directing that love to your baby, surrounding the womb with love, imagine this love to be a soothing pastel light that envelopes your baby.* [PAUSE.] *Now say quietly in your own mind and direct your statements to your baby, "I love you and I am* [OR *"we are"*] *anxious for your arrival."* [PAUSE.] *Now say quietly in your mind, "You are wanted."* [PAUSE.] *Again, "You are wanted."* [PAUSE.] *Now just imagine that your baby is smiling and that he or she has received your message. Continue to relax, relax your body. As you continue to relax, imagine the birth day arriving . . .* [IN-SERT THE APPROPRIATE TIME, BASED ON YOUR DUE DATE. FOR EXAMPLE, "six months from now," "June 17th," OR "tomorrow."] *You feel the first hints of labor and it is easy for you to apply the lessons in proper breathing and muscle control. You are calm and relaxed, breathing correctly; whenever you feel discomfort you take your thoughts far away to your special place, you breathe evenly, you know exactly what needs to be done. Whenever you feel discomfort, you know what needs to be done, exactly what needs to be done. Imagine giving birth, pushing when you need to, breathing properly and feeling comfortable, your mind is far away in your special place, you experience the birth process, you feel yourself push and breathe and you feel comfortable, in charge, relaxed. You are comfortable, in control, relaxed; you are comfortable, in control, relaxed. Your delivery is successful in every way, in every way, and when the baby arrives it is healthy and strong, it is healthy and strong.* [PAUSE.] *Now imagine yourself home with your baby, you are a natural mother, you know instinctively how to care for your child. You are enjoying motherhood, you accept the changes in your life with enthusiasm, you see difficulties as challenges and are able to meet your needs as well as the family's needs. Just see yourself smiling, feeling good about yourself and your life and see yourself as the attractive, capable and loving woman you are.* [PAUSE.] *See yourself smiling, feeling good about yourself and your life, and see yourself as the attractive, capable, and loving woman you are.* [PAUSE.] *See yourself smiling, feeling good about yourself and your life, and see yourself as the attractive, capable, and loving woman you are. Now just relax in your special place for another moment and soon you can begin to return to full consciousness, feeling relaxed and refreshed.*

What You Can Expect

With proper preparation and training, you can expect to enjoy a healthy pregnancy, control in labor and delivery, and a reduction or elimination of pain. After the birth, you will find yourself in good spirits with a positive attitude. In the case below, Laura experienced all of the positive elements of childbirth, as they have been discussed in the preceding material.

Case Study

Laura, 26, and Cameron, 30, were expecting their second child. Laura's first birthing experience had been painful. She had a difficult labor and delivery, so she believed that the second birth would be an equally painful experience. She hoped hypnosis would help her support and reinforce her natural childbirth training as well as reduce and eliminate pain. Throughout her pregnancy, Laura practiced the *Relaxation Induction,* using positive imagery and the *Childbirth Induction.* In addition, she did the Lamaze breathing and relaxation exercises, which included muscle control.

When the day of delivery arrived and Laura felt the first signs of labor, she began her breathing exercises. Her husband served as her coach, reinforcing and reminding her of her proper breathing and relaxation techniques. When she arrived at the hospital and was escorted into the delivery room, her mind was already in the special place she had used in her *Childbirth Induction* for seven months. Her chosen place was a forest on the Olympic peninsula in Washington.

Laura felt no discomfort during delivery. She was in control, breathing, pushing, relaxing. One part of her mind was busily engaged in the birthing process, while another part—the part that registers pain—was far away sitting on a blanket in the sunlit forest where she had once spent a wonderful vacation.

At one point, Laura was so relaxed that the obstetrician had to request that she return from her trance state to push with the contractions. She obliged and felt no discomfort.

Before delivery, Laura had often imagined speaking to the baby and telling it to hurry and come quickly because her husband couldn't wait for its arrival. She told the baby that they loved it and were eager to hold it. Apparently the baby got the message, because she arrived on time and the labor was short. Laura delivered a healthy little girl. In the recovery room, Cameron played a tape of soft music before they had a champagne toast to Lisa Marie.

9

Health Problems

Allen consumes a large meal in eight minutes, settles in front of his TV, lights up a cigarette, pours himself a drink, and relaxes. In a few moments he experiences a sharp pain in his chest. He has felt this pain on and off for several months. His doctor has diagnosed the condition as the beginning stages of heart disease. Allen had anticipated this information, since his father suffered from the same condition. Allen believes he can do nothing for his problem and continues his destructive life style.

Kathy arrives at work 15 minutes late. She has a slight headache and is a bit nauseated. She resists the idea of going home because there is an important sales meeting in the afternoon. But, as noon approaches, she becomes increasingly ill and is forced to leave the office. That evening, she recovers completely. The following week, Kathy is scheduled to give a presentation to a group of co-workers at 3:30. At 1:30 she develops an asthma attack and has to go home. She visits her doctor, who can find no asthmatic condition.

Dean awakens in the morning with a painful sensation that extends from his ear to the base of his neck. He finds it impossible to turn his head from side to side. After two weeks of intermittent bouts with the discomfort, Dean visits his doctor, who can't find anything wrong and suggests that heat and massage will help. Dean follows the doctor's recommendations and gets some relief, but the tightness and pain often reoccur over the next few months, and each time the condition lasts for days. Dean decides that his condition is chronic and he will have to learn to live with it.

These three people are similar in the following ways: (1) they all suffer from ill health, (2) they have little or no understanding of the cause of their condition, and (3) they exercise no control over their own health.

Allen, Kathy, and Dean need to gain a clear understanding of their physical and mental states. As they discover the causes of their illnesses and the options and techniques available to them, they will be better equipped to gain control over their own health and general well-being.

Major Causes of Health Problems

As mysterious as the onset of any of your health problems may seem to be, the general causes are usually quite clear-cut. Most health problems evolve from one of the three following situations.

Your health problems may be caused by stress. Because stress is very often a major component of contemporary life, the word itself has become part of our everyday vocabulary: "The stress in our relationship is ruining our marriage." "His stress level is so high, he's ready to explode." "I don't mind the work itself, it's the stress that's getting me down."

No one is immune to stress. But when stress becomes a persistent negative factor in your life, it can cause a collapse of your body's defenses, which, in turn, cause a breakdown in your resistance to illness, disease, chronic conditions, or mental disorders.

Stressful situations produce reactions that can manifest themselves differently from one individual to another, and even from one gender to another. For example, studies have shown that given an identical stress stimulus, men and women will have differing physiological reactions. For example, it has been proven that the mere activity of talking to someone causes a stress response: In men, the blood pressure becomes elevated, and in women the blood pressure does not change as much as the heart rate.

Of course, the severity of a stress reaction varies in accordance with the stimulus. A stimulus may be as minor as talking to someone in a position of superiority, or it may be a major trauma, such as the death of a spouse. A "stress scale" has been developed by Thomas H. Holmes, a doctor at the University of Washington School of Medicine in Seattle. This scale establishes the relationship between significant events in a person's life and physical or emotional disorders.

To give you an example of how these events rank, the death of a spouse has a mean value of 100, a divorce 73, a marital separation

65, retirement 45, pregnancy 40, sexual difficulties 39, changing to a new school 20, and a vacation 13. Of those people who have a score exceeding 300 for the past year, almost 80 percent become ill in the near future; with a score of 150 to 299, about 50 percent become ill in the near future; and with a score of less than 150, only about 30 percent become ill. So the more life changes you experience, the harder you need to work to stay well.

When a person's life change is accompanied by leisure time, the individual has more hours in the day to concentrate on his or her physical condition. People who retire and women who worked maintaining a home for children who have departed for work or college often have health problems of two general types: (1) problems that had been previously overlooked or consciously ignored due to a life style that was "outwardly focused," and (2) problems that are the product of newly-created personal anxieties.

Your environment and your body are major culprits in the stress syndrome. External conditions in the environment that you may not recognize as stress stimuli can wreak their own havoc. These may include frequent exposure to crowds, exposure to danger, unsatisfactory domestic living conditions, undesirable weather, or noise.

These environmental conditions are often made worse by your attitudes or beliefs about them. For example, a study was done of residents living near Heathrow Airport in London and Kennedy Airport in New York. The residents who assumed that the pilots, airport personnel, and government officials didn't care about the inconvenience and disturbance of airport noise were extremely annoyed. Further, those who thought the noise was not necessary, that it was threatening to their health, or that they were in the path of potential plane crashes, were additionally stressed. In direct contrast, those residents who believed that someone cared about the noise and was trying to deal with it were less stressed by it.

Those stresses which result from the body, from physiological sources, are of two kinds: avoidable and unavoidable. In the avoidable category are those that are the result of such conditions as poor diet or insomnia. Those in the unavoidable category include such conditions as aging or adolescence.

Regardless of the type of stress your body is undergoing, the physical ailments that may result are many and varied: headaches, peptic ulcers, arthritis, colitis, diarrhea, asthma, cardiac arhythmia, sexual problems, circulatory problems, muscle tension, and even cancer.

In *The Stress of Life,* Hans Selye asserts that the basis for all illness and disease is stress. There are those who would feel this is an overstatement. But it is certainly true that any predisposition to illness or disease is intensified by stress—even if the stress itself does not seem to be directly identified with the cause.

Chronic conditions that result from stress can often be very unique and elusive. This was true for Ethel, a 62-year-old homemaker who for two years had experienced spasms in the muscles around her eyes and eyelids that produced an involuntary closure of her eyes. Even though Ethel was not narcoleptic, she had her eyes closed most of the time.

When the spasms began, her eyelids would shut tightly. The hypnotherapist noticed that Ethel's eyelids *did* open when she was engaged in conversation, but only when she was speaking. As long as she talked, her eyes stayed open. Ethel was not aware of this and thought that her eyelids opened only sporadically. Medical consultations had netted only two alternatives for Ethel. Her eyelids could be sewn up to keep them open and drops used to provide the necessary moisture for the eye, or the nerves could be deadened. Hypnosis was sought in the hope that it would keep Ethel from having to accept these medical alternatives. The program that was designed for Ethel consisted of the *Stress Reduction Induction,* the *Relaxation Induction,* and a posthypnotic suggestion that included positive imagery. The induction suggested, "Each day your eyes will stay open for longer and longer periods of time." As Ethel entered the hypnotic trance, she was instructed to speak in her normal voice and tell about something she enjoyed doing (one of her talents or skills) in great detail. As Ethel told a story about one of her greatest accomplishments, embroidering costumes for a ten-member contemporary dance troupe, she enjoyed recounting her great achievement.

As Ethel was speaking, the hypnotherapist suggested that Ethel continue to relax. Ethel easily entered a trance state with her eyes open while engaging in conversation. As the induction progressed, the hypnotherapist instructed Ethel to lower her voice. She complied, and each time the suggestion was given, her eyes continued to stay open. Soon she was whispering with her eyes open. Finally, she was merely mouthing the words, using no audible speech at all. Her eyes continued to stay open. In that state, a posthypnotic suggestion was given that explained, "Since your eyes are open and since you are not uttering a sound, your eyes will now continue to stay open even when you are not speaking and your eyes will stay open for longer and longer periods each day."

The sessions were given twice weekly over a six-week period. In the third week, Ethel noticed tremendous progress. Her eyes stayed open for an entire day for the first time in two years. But the next day her eyes shut tightly for the entire day. This lapse was a product of temporary resistance because, to some degree, Ethel wanted to continue to shut out the world. Continued suggestions of relaxation, self-esteem, and positive imagery were given for the remainder of the six-week period. On completion, Ethel's eyes stayed open, and she was able to resume a normal daily life. It was recommended that Ethel seek psychotherapy to gain a better understanding of the source of her stress and why it affected her so dramatically.

Your health problem may be inherited. Certain familiar illnesses, such as allergies, asthma, diabetes, and heart disease, may be inherited. That is, you may be predisposed to these conditions. There are three courses this type of health problem can take: (1) It may manifest itself at a relatively early age, or even at birth. (2) It may become evident during a period of extreme stress due to a dramatic change in your life pattern or during a time of difficult and prolonged personal demands. (3) It may remain as a dormant condition throughout your entire life.

If your inherited health problem takes the third course, you have no need to worry. However, if you became the victim of an inherited illness or disease at birth or during your childhood, you can take action to combat or perhaps even alleviate the symptoms of your health problem. Similarly, if the problem surfaced at a time of extreme stress, you can first treat the stress and then focus on the specific symptom or condition.

Jane, an investment broker, is a daughter and granddaughter of women who had been the victims of breast cancer. When Jane was 40 and recently divorced, she discovered a small tumor in her breast. She was successfully treated with chemotherapy and her cancer went into remission.

Fortunately, Jane was convinced that her own mental attitude could affect changes in her body. She was determined to reduce the stress she was experiencing as a result of the divorce, having two teenage children, and increased pressure at work. She made a pact with herself and her hypnotherapist to participate fully in her own health care. Jane used the *Stress Reduction Induction* and the *General Healing Induction* in this chapter. She also created her own positive imagery, which she incorporated into the *General Healing Induction*. This imagery suggested that silky soft scrub brushes were cleaning and scrubbing away any cancer in her breasts. She used her induction every other day for the first two weeks, then twice a week for a period of eight weeks. She has remained free of cancer for the past eight years.

Your health problem may be the result of an injury or an accident. When suffering from the shock produced by an injury or accident, your body reacts in a variety of ways. Three of the major reactions are (1) lower blood pressure, (2) a diminished pulse rate, and (3) a temperature below normal. In extreme cases, the shock can result in death. In all cases, the shock of accident or injury produces a breakdown of the body's defenses. Specifically, shock is a depression or cessation of the influences of the nervous system over various important bodily functions, principally the circulation and respiration. The results vary in intensity, depending on the patient and the injury.

Therefore, the effect may be temporary or it may linger, resulting in a chronic condition. In this state, your immune system is weakened, and you are more prone to illness or geneanl health problems. For example, some people become allergic to things that previously had not produced any allergic reaction at all.

Of course, you can also experience illness, disease, or chronic disorders as a *direct* result of an injury or accident. These problems may include back spasms, arthritic conditions in the injured joints, tendonitis, numbness, tingling, cardiac arhythmia, colitis, or respiratory problems.

Dave, a 27-year-old ex-surfer, was injured when he fell from a painting scaffold. He was hospitalized briefly for back injuries from which he recovered.

Before Dave's accident, he had never experienced any muscle spasms. However, in the year following the accident he became temporarily disabled six times by muscle spasms in his back. Each time these occurred, Dave took muscle relaxants and pain killers for three or four days until he could return to work.

In his first interview with the hypnotherapist, she suspected from his gait that Dave might be pampering his back; that is, his posture had been adjusted to compensate for what he still perceived as a back injury. Dave was also an intense individual who seemed to internalize his problems. His treatment conisted of a *Stress Reduction Induction* and a specific healing suggestion that focused on his back, spine, and posture. The *General Healing Induction* in this chapter was also included. During the induction, it was suggested to Dave that he had a strong, pliant back which allowed him to have erect posture and to perform in his job of painting contractor. He was told, "You can do your work well because you trust your back and you have good muscle tone, stamina, and strength."

Along with the hypnotherapy, Dave did some exercises that were recommended by his doctor for strengthening back muscles. Within weeks, Dave said that he felt a change in his overall health. To date, he has not had any reoccurring bouts with muscle spasms, and it has been two years since he used his program of hypnotherapy and physical exercises. He is now engaging in sports again and swims regularly at a health spa. He says that he feels better than he did before the accident.

Your health problem may be HIV/AIDS related. HIV (Human Immunodeficiency Virus) is the virus that can cause AIDS (Acquired Immune Deficiency Syndrome). HIV destroys certain cells in the body, weakening the immune system and causing a person to be defenseless against opportunistic infections such as:

- Kaposi's sarcoma (KS): A type of skin cancer.
- Pneumocystis carinii pneumonia (PCP): A form of pneumonia.

- Shingles: An acute infection that causes painful blisters on the skin.
- Tuberculosis: A communicable disease that primarily affects the lungs, but can affect any part of the body.

Studies show emotions have a tremendous impact on the immune system. Fear, anger, depression, and stress take their toll both emotionally and physically. These feelings are to be expected since the HIV/AIDS infected person faces many complex issues.

Jerry and Mark have AIDS and have been combating various opportunistic infections for over seven years. They both attribute their continual survival to having a positive attitude and keeping stress to a minimum. Hypnotherapy was suggested to them as a means of reducing stress and boosting their immune systems.

The hypnotherapy sessions were given simultaneously to both Jerry and Mark once a week for a six-week period. In certain situations, receiving hypnosis together can be a very supportive approach. The program began with the *Stress Reduction Induction* followed by the *General Healing Induction*. During the course of the program, Jerry and Mark were encouraged to design posthypnotic suggestions specific to their particular needs. In addition, the hypnotherapist created imagery to boost the function of their immune system, which she incorporated into the *General Healing Induction*. This imagery suggested visualizing what the immune system looks like. Once visualized, they were told to imagine healing cells flowing through their immune system, strengthening and boosting the power of their immune system. The inductions were recorded at each session and practiced daily. In the first few weeks, both Jerry and Mark reported feeling more relaxed. By the end of their six week program, each felt that the inductions (along with imagery boosting the immune system) helped them to reduce stress and maintain a positive attitude.

Your health problem may result from cancer treatment. Hypnosis can be utilized for the many phases of cancer treatment. Symptoms of the disease range from deep emotional distress to pain caused by medical treatments and surgery. Hypnosis can be applied to help manage the pain associated with specific organs, fatigue, irritability, low blood count, infection, insomnia, and side effects of chemotherapy and radiation, such as nausea and vomiting.

Suggestions given during the hypnotic trance can change the sensation of pain from intense to a more manageable state, sometimes eliminating it altogether. However, because pain is an important indicator that can help determine the course of medical treatment, care must be given before eliminating pain altogether. Another suggestion for pain management can include placing the pain far away to distance the patient from the discomfort.

The deep relaxing that occurs during the hypnotic induction may automatically reduce fatigue, irritability, and insomnia. Twenty minutes of hypnotic relaxation can equal one to two hours of sleep. Coupling with specific suggestions such as "feeling calm and relaxed, and sleeping soundly" will produce quick results. (Refer to Chapter 15 for more on insomnia.)

The autonomic nervous system is responsible for controlling involuntary body functions, such as sweating, digestion, and heart rate. Hypnotic suggestions help these functions to relax, calming heart rate and aiding digestion.

Mental imagery of a normal blood count and healthy cells may strengthen the immune system to fight infection. Visualizing red and white blood cells surging through the body with healthy, powerful cells fighting the infection can be used in both the pre- or postsurgery phase.

Setting Up Your Plan of a Lifetime

Regardless of the specific nature of your health problem, your major goal will be one of these two: (1) to reduce discomfort and pain of a chronic condition or (2) to heal and recover quickly and to maintain good health.

These objectives can be achieved only through the careful construction of a sound (or improved) health platform from which to operate. This platform includes the following:

1. Good nutrition
2. The elimination of harmful substances, including cigarettes, alcohol, toxic substances in your environment, and prescriptive drugs that are no longer necessary
3. The reduction of stimulants
4. Improved personal safety
5. Early detection of illness; self-examination and awareness of bodily changes
6. Reduction of stressful situations and negative conditions in your life
7. Periodic leisure time, scheduled as necessary

Programming for Results

The inductions in this chapter are designed to help you think, feel, and act in certain ways. They program your subconscious by offering logical and realistic suggestions, as well as imaginative positive suggestions that include imagery. Below are the specific objectives necessary to gain control over your health and to incorporate new behavior.

Practice relaxation to reduce stress. The *Relaxation Induction*, which is one component of the total *Health Induction*, suggests, "Release any tension, any stress from any part of your body, mind, and thought; just let that stress go. Just feel any stressful thoughts rushing through your mind, feel them begin to wind down, wind down, wind down, and relax. Notice how very comfortable your body feels, just drifting and floating, deeper, deeper, deeper relaxed . . ."

Visualize and focus on positive images that counteract your specific illness or condition. The imagery you use will depend on your specific health problem. The *Treating Your Health Problems* section in this chapter includes numerous suggestions to use within your major induction. For example, if cancer is your specific health problem, you can suggest, "Focus your attention on the area of your cancer, now imagine what your cancer might look like, you can imagine it to be anything you like, it may be a school of little fish that get eaten up by very large and ferocious fish. You can use any image, the color red that changes to blue is fine, and when the red is all replaced by blue and the red is gone, the cancer is gone, completely gone. And now imagine it shriveling and drying up, shrinking, shrinking away to the size of a pinpoint as you rid yourself of this intruder. The cells are whole and healthy, completely whole and healthy and your healing process has worked."

Visualize and focus on positive images that augment general and total healing. The *General Healing Induction,* which is one of the components of your total *Health Induction,* suggests, "Breathe deeply. And now just imagine a healing white light begin at the top of your head and surround your entire body, feel its velvet softness on your skin, this white light is healing, soothing, and calming. Just feel it surround your entire body, see it on the surface of your skin, and now just feel it soak into your body. Feel it circulate throughout your entire body, healing and cleansing every organ, nerve, muscle, and cell of your body. Feel its gentle warmth flow through your head, across your eyes, melt down your shoulders . . ."

Program your subconscious to maintain good health. The *General Healing Induction* suggests, "Now imagine yourself, healthy and strong, vibrant. There's a smile on your face, you feel wonderful, healthy and strong, healthy and strong. This positive image will grow stronger and stronger every day."

Your Treatment Plan

You will need to use two major inductions, each consisting of several components. The first major induction will be used when you are experiencing the discomfort that is associated with your specific health problem. The second induction can be used at any time to promote general healing and a healthy body.

To record the first induction, follow the directions for items 1, 2, and 4 below. To record the second induction for general healing, follow the directions for items 1, 3, and 4 below.

1. Turn to Chapter 2 and use the *Going Down Induction*.

2. Look at the *Treating Your Health Problems* section of this chapter. Find the health problem you need to eliminate. Next, read the suggestion for your specific problem. Following the directions below, personalize your suggestion and record it immediately following the *Going Down Induction*. As you record, you should repeat the key phrases within the suggestion, then repeat the whole suggestion a second time.

3. Immediately following the *Going Down Induction*, record the *General Healing Induction* in this chapter.

4. Close with the *Coming Up Induction* from Chapter 2.

These components should be recorded so that they flow together to make two total health inductions. They will work together to meet your individual needs. Item 1 provides relaxation. Item 2 deals with your specific health problem. Item 3 promotes healing to produce a totally healthy body. Item 4 brings you out of the induction in a relaxed and pleasant state.

The suggestions in the *Treating Your Health Problems* section are presented there as models. You should expand upon the theme of the suggestions you select; that is, it can serve as a core, around which you build a thoroughly effective posthypnotic induction. *What* you insert into this suggestion or add to it is determined by the particular characteristics of your specific health problem. As you develop a personalized suggestion, remember to employ the key components of an effective suggestion as explained in Chapter 2. Use *synonyms* for reinforcement, *paraphrase your suggestions, use connective words* to maintain a steady flow of language, and *designate time* ("in just a few moments," "now you will," and so on) when you need to signal the beginning or end of a particular behavior. (Note: If your health problem is not included in this section, find one that is similar to yours and read the suggestion for the problem. Then, using it as a model, write your own suggestion by referring to the *Guidelines for Effective Suggestions* in Chapter 3.)

TREATING YOUR HEALTH PROBLEM

Follow the guidelines provided in the *Your Treatment Plan* section in this chapter to personalize and record the specific posthypnotic suggestion for your health problem.

ALLERGIES

Take a deep breath and begin to breathe more easily. [PAUSE.] *Take another deep breath and feel your sinuses open* [PAUSE], *air passing through them and down into your lungs, exhale and feel any tension leave your body.* [PAUSE.] *Imagine yourself breathing clean fresh air, the kind of clean fresh air you might experience on a snowy mountain top or by a beautiful ocean, so refreshing, so exhilarating, so easy to breathe, cooling and fresh, from now, on whenever you see or feel the substance you are allergic to just imagine the snowy mountain or the wide cool ocean and relax your breathing, breathe slowly and feel your sinuses open, accepting air easily through them, breathing easily, feeling so relaxed, breathing clean, fresh air.* [REPEAT.]

ASTHMA AND BRONCHIAL CONDITIONS

Relax and breathe slowly and evenly [PAUSE], *breathe slowly and evenly* [PAUSE], *feel the air pass easily through your nostrils, down your windpipe and into your lungs* [PAUSE], *you are in control of your breathing, complete control, from now on whenever you feel an asthmatic surge begin you can quickly stop it by relaxing every muscle in your body. Concentrate on your breathing, relax your breathing, and begin to imagine yourself in a beautiful clear desert, breathing in clear autumn air, feeling it go deep into your lungs. As you imagine this clear desert air going deep into your lungs, your breathing returns to normal, returns to normal.* [REPEAT.]

BOOSTING THE IMMUNE SYSTEM

As you relax more and more, begin to imagine your immune system, it can be any image that you want, it can be any shape, size, color, or object, whatever comes into mind. Let this image become more clear and more detailed. There are many functions that contribute to a healthy immune system, some of them involve healthy blood cells, others include the function of certain glands. And all you need to do is to imagine that all systems are working perfectly to boost your immunity system. Just like a fine tuned instrument, every system in your body is working efficiently to boost the power of your immune system. Now imagine your immune system responding in the most positive way, see it become stronger, protecting your body, protecting every function of your body. Now just imagine your immune system growing stronger and stronger, more powerful, functioning at peak performance. [REPEAT.]

CANCER

Focus your attention on the area of your cancer, now imagine how your cancer might look, you can imagine it to be anything you like, it may be a school of little fish that get eaten up by a very large and ferocious fish, or it can be the angry color red that changes to a calm, quiet blue. You can use any image you like, any image is just fine. [PAUSE.] *Now just imagine the cancer drying up, shrinking, shrinking to the size of a pinpoint. The cancer disappears somewhere far off in the distance where no one can find it, far, far off in the distance. Begin to imagine your cells whole and healthy and your healing process has worked, you are healing, growing stronger, stronger, becoming healthy once again.* [REPEAT.]

CARDIOVASCULAR DISORDERS

Relax your chest, inhale, and as you inhale focus your attention on the rhythm of your heart [PAUSE], *exhale slowly* [PAUSE], *and feel the rhythm, calm, even, and relaxed, just imagine the even flow of your blood through your veins and arteries, your heart muscle pumping and working perfectly, with every beat, your heart muscle strengthens, becomes strong and vibrant, just feel the even and calm rhythm of your strong heart, calm and even, calm and even. Your heart is strong and dependable and works exactly as it should. The rhythm of your heart is even, even, calm, strong, and your heart is strong.* [REPEAT.]

COLDS AND FLU

As you relax, set aside any feelings of discomfort and concentrate on total relaxation, health and healing, begin to imagine your entire body filled from the toes up to the top of your head with the color orange, just like a glass of orange juice. Now imagine that you pull a plug out from the bottom of your feet and imagine all of the orange color drain slowly out of your body, as it drains out of your body it takes with it all infections, flu bugs and any substances that are harmful to your health, feel it drain away, just as if you were slowly pouring out a glass of orange juice, just feel it drain away, drain away, once you have completely drained the orange color from the top of your head to your toes, fill your body up from your toes to the top of your head with a soft golden color that heals your body and restores new healthy energy Now just feel the golden color, heal, heal, and feel a new and vibrant energy fill your body. [REPEAT.]

COLITIS

Feel the muscles in your abdomen relax, focus your attention on your abdomen and feel a soothing warmth flow through your lower in-

testinal region, just below your navel, imagine a warm healing sensation flowing through your intestines, your organs, and into your colon, soothing and relaxing, soothing and relaxing. You can think of your intestinal region as new, completely new, and healthy and working perfectly, calmly, slowly, and you are in control of it, complete control [REPEAT]

HIGH BLOOD PRESSURE

Relax and begin to imagine what your normal blood pressure should be [INSERT NUMBERS.] *You imagine your blood pressure to be normal, completely normal, if you are on medication for your blood pressure, then just imagine the medication working effectively and quickly. If your high blood pressure is due to stress, then begin to imagine your stressful situation change because you change your reaction to the stimulus, imagine yourself calm and relaxed, with your blood pressure normal throughout any stressful situation, now just imagine once again what your blood pressure should be.* [INSERT NUMBERS.] *Imagine your blood pressure normal, imagine yourself calm and relaxed, feeling healthy and strong, rejecting harmful stress, enjoying your life, feeling calm and relaxed, calm and relaxed.* [SEE CHAPTER 6 FOR MORE SPECIFIC TREATMENT FOR SEVERE STRESS.]

TENSION

Feel yourself relax, know that you are in control of your choices, you have the choice to be stressed, nervous, or easily upset, you also have the choice to be calm, relaxed, and at ease with your environment, and you now choose to experience life in a calm and relaxed way and to flow easily with its ups and downs. Imagine some of your stressful situations and imagine that you now react to them in a calm and relaxed manner, your stomach is relaxed, you breathe easily and evenly, if you imagine yourself among people, then imagine yourself at ease, your conversation is flowing smoothly, you are calm and relaxed. At work the pressure may mount but you stay calm, at ease and relaxed, your stomach is calm, you breathe easily and evenly, from now on you will make the choice to relax in any situation, you will feel yourself breathing easily and evenly, now just let this new choice for peace and calm flow through every cell of your body. [REPEAT. SEE CHAPTER 6 FOR MORE SPECIFIC TREATMENT FOR SEVERE STRESS.]

MIGRAINE HEADACHES

Feel the muscles in your temples relax, focus your attention on the muscles across your forehead and feel those muscles relax, rest your eyes and inhale deeply. [PAUSE.] *Exhale and feel all the muscles in your head relax.* [PAUSE.] *Now follow the muscles across your forehead, focus on those muscles, across your forehead, around your head, over your ears and to the base of the skull, and relax this area, relax the area as you go across your forehead, around your head over your ears and to the base of your neck, imagine a cool breeze blowing across your face, cooling your head, your face, your eyes. Imagine a cool and soothing sensation across your forehead and above each eye. Imagine walking along a snowy path in the mountains. Your hands are tucked in your pockets, they are warm, they are warm. Your hands are warm and comfortable, while a cool breeze and cold air makes your head feel cooler, soothing and relaxing every muscle, releasing any tightness, any stress. Just feel a calm sensation flow through your eyes and forehead, you are calm and comfortable and relaxed.* [REPEAT.]

[NOTE: The warming of the hands during this suggestion is important. When the blood vessels of the hands are dilated, the pressure is reduced in the enlarged blood vessels in the head.]

MUSCLE SPASMS

Focus your attention on the muscle that is tight and strained, now relax the muscle that is stressed, relax it and let your mind concentrate on the muscle and think about relaxing that muscle, as you think about relaxing that muscle begin to feel it relax, relax the muscles and nerves around the area when you feel discomfort, just imagine a comfortable heating pad, soothing and warming and relaxing the area. [INSERT THE AREA WHERE THE MUSCLE SPASM IS LOCATED.] *Feel all tension and tightness drain away from the muscle, as if you were releasing the air from a balloon and all of the strain is released and soon the balloon is limp, limp and pliable, just as your strained muscle is when you release and relax that muscle, limp and relaxed, limp and relaxed, and as you relax this muscle soon this area will regain vibrant and healthy energy, strength and power, now just feel your muscle soothed and relaxed.* [REPEAT.]

STOMACH DISORDERS

Inhale deeply [PAUSE] *and exhale slowly and as you exhale slowly feel your stomach relax.* [PAUSE.] *Relax all the muscles around your stomach area. With every even breatth you take, feel your stomach relax more and more. Now tell your subconscious to keep this area stress-free, your stomach will now digest food properly and maintain perfect function, feel your stomach relax, whenever you are in a stressful situation, relax your stomach, imagine a soothing sensation, calming the surface of your stomach, calming your stomach, just feel your stomach relax, relax, calm and relaxed.* [REPEAT]

PEPTIC ULCER

Relax, relax every muscle, relax, now just imagine taking all of your worries and problems and placing them in a shoe box, you put the lid on the box and you take the box to your closet and place it on the top shelf. [PAUSE.] *You can always retrieve it later if you need to, but for now those worries are put away and you enjoy being free of them, now just release all the stress from your body, mind and emotions, feel a sense of peace and calm wrap around your body forming a protective shield, shielding you from any excessive stress at work, home, or any situation that may be stressful to you. You are now protected, stress just bounces off and away from you, you feel a calm flow through your body, its pleasant warm sensation, feel it now enter your stomach region, feel it smooth and heal your ulcer, soothe and calm, and because you are calm and at peace, your ulcer will heal quickly, your subconscious is now programmed to keep your stomach stress-free and to reject negative stress from your body, mind, and emotions, and as you continue to enjoy this peaceful feeling you will regain new and healthy energy, and now continue to relax, feeling a pleasant calm flow through your body, healing, healing, calming, calming.* [REPEAT.]

GENERAL HEALING INDUCTION

Breathe deeply and evenly, let your mind and body rest, set aside all cares, set aside all cares, and think only of total relaxation, total complete relaxation, and now just imagine a healing white light at the top of your head. It spreads out and surrounds your entire body, surrounds your entire body, see it on the surface of your skin and now feel it circulate throughout your body, throughout your entire body, healing and cleansing, healing and cleansing every inch of your body, every organ, nerve, muscle, and cell of your body, every organ, nerve, muscle, and cell of your body, feel it circulate throughout your body, and now feel its gentle warmth flow through your head, feel it flow through your head, through your head and across your eyes, feel it melt down to your shoulders, circulating around your neck and down your back, now up your back again into your shoulders and down to your chest, feel it circulate around your heart, through your lungs and into your stomach, through your intestines, cleansing and healing, cleansing and healing, over and over again, it is cleansing and healing your whole body. Now imagine yourself healthy and strong, healthy and strong and vibrant. There's a smile on your face, you feel wonderful, healthy and strong, healthy and strong, and this positive image will grow stronger and stronger every day.

What to Expect and Following Up

Use your induction with the specific suggestion for treating your health problem whenever you feel discomfort and need relief. Use the *General*

Healing Induction every day for the first week and three times a week for the next two or three weeks. When you notice positive changes occurring, you may return to using the *General Healing Induction* every day for a week. Then gradually cut back until the symptoms are gone (or reduced to such a degree that your level of discomfort is minimal). The frequency level fluctuates in order to allow time for your subconscious to accept and respond to suggestion. If you suddenly and continually bombard your subconscious without giving it any assimilation time, your chances of experiencing improved health may be reduced.

Special Considerations

In 1984 it was estimated that approximately 15,000 doctors, dentists, psychologists, and other health-care workers used hypnosis in their clinical practices. And it is important to recognize that hypnosis is gaining acceptance as a method of treatment. But it is still necessary for you to *consult with your doctor about your specific health problem before you begin to use hypnotherapy.*

Further, you must keep in mind that your total health program consists of many elements and that those elements, as outlined in the preceding material, work together to help you deal with your health problems. You can use hypnotherapy for twenty years, but if you smoke three packs of cigarettes a day and never get any exercise, you're not going to have an easy time reducing the symptoms of your chronic bronchitis. Remember that hypnosis cannot function in isolation, but must be an adjunctive form of treatment, rather than a sole alternative.

10

Pain Control

Surrounded by redwoods and cooled by the breeze of a June night, a group of 70 people have gathered under the stars in a small mountain community. At first glance, they could easily be mistaken for a group of campers, ending their day with a visit around the campfire. But this is not the case. These people have gathered around a bed of glowing coals that many of them will walk on before the night is over.

This group and many others like it consist of "firewalkers" who are able to enter a state that allows them to walk over coals, ranging in temperature from 600 to 1200 degrees. The majority of them will experience no discomfort.

Though the conditions that allow a successful walk are described and explained in a variety of ways, they all have one element in common: the trance state. This state does not differ significantly from the hypnotic state experienced by shamans in primitive cultures. Many of the components of the experience are the same. They include careful preparation, chanting, the use of a key word or phrase, and visualizing.

On this particular night in northern California, a number of people in the group—among them students, a medical technologist, a retired senior citizen, and an English professor—walk across the fire and out, wiping their feet on the turf to remove any embers from their skin before they emerge from their trance state.

This experience is not recounted to encourage you to become a firewalker. It is, however, a dramatic and very real example of the degree to which a person can use his or her mind to control or prohibit painful sensations.

Pain: Its Origins and Accomplices

You know pain as a physical sensation that causes bodily suffering and distress. To understand exactly how this physical pain is sensed, imagine this: You are standing in a crowd. The person in front of you backs up and tromps on your toe. Several chemical substances that are stored near your nerve endings are released. These chemicals make the nerve endings sensitive, so that the pain message can be transmitted from the toe to the brain. These chemicals also increase circulation to the injured area, which then causes swelling and redness. This process is a natural one that augments healing and fights off bacteria.

The pain message then travels to the spinal cord, on to the sensory center of the brain, and to the cortex where the location of the pain is deciphered. It is at this point that you say to yourself (or scream aloud), "Ouch, you clumsy fool. You've stepped on my toe!"

Then you get some help. Chemicals that provide pain relief are released in the brain and spinal cord, and the pain in your toe seems less severe than it was moments ago.

This example illustrates a pain resulting from injury. However, the basic pain process is the same, regardless of the stimulant. The painful sensations may come from a wide range of causes—from chronic condition to debilitating disease—but the path the pain takes is still the same, as are the basic physiological reactions to it.

Not to be overlooked in considering pain's impact and its intensity are four other factors: your emotions, your previous experiences or associations with pain, your characteristics, and your perception of what the pain signifies to you. Each one of these factors is worth a brief examination.

Your emotions. When you experience pain as a result of illness, disease, or a chronic condition (as opposed to a temporary pain, such as that of a pinched finger), the anxiety and the pain itself are inseparable. Depending on your particular situation, your anxiety may be even more severe than the pain. Those who suffer from chronic pain often are the victims of a resulting cycle of emotional and physical symptoms: anxiety, depression, loss of appetite, extreme fatigue, and insomnia. Pain continues to perpetuate the cycle and the result is often complete debilitation due to these byproducts of pain.

Narrowing this focus slightly, a study of emotional reactions among cancer patients revealed dread of continued pain, despair, unhappiness due to changes in self-image, uncertainty, depression, and fear—of being completely incapacitated, of financial destitution, isolation, or death.

Just as pain can bring forth emotions, emotions can summon pain. Pain can sometimes be brought into being as a means of preventing oneself from becoming aggressive and hostile. Pain has also been linked with guilt, which may either exist because of current behavior or be the outgrowth of a problem that is deeply rooted in the past. For example, pain can serve as a self-imposed penance for sexual pleasures which the pain victim sees as "bad" or unconventional. It is important to note, however, that psychological origins are not associated with the majority of pain victims.

Your previous experiences or associations with pain. It has been shown that people often react to pain in accordance with general patterns established in childhood or, to some degree, ethnic tradition. Two rather isolated studies substantiate this point. In the first, children from larger families tended to be more verbal about their pain than children from families with fewer children. It may be that the children with several siblings felt they needed to voice their distress loud and clear in order to get the attention they felt the situation deserved. The second example arises from a study done with Yankees ("old Americans"), Irish, Jews, and Italians. The groups predisposed to overt behavioral responses to pain were Jews and Italian women, both representatives of groups who do not disapprove of overt reactions.

Similarly, people whose role models react to pain in a certain way will be likely to copy this behavior themselves. Just as you can "acquire" a phobia by observing someone else's fear (of elevators, spiders, bridges), you can also acquire a response to pain.

If you associate pain with something pleasant, it is likely to be less severe than if it is associated with a negative factor or outcome. For example, if you think your pain indicates that a disease that you had thought yourself free of has returned, you are likely to experience pain of a greater intensity than if you knew the pain to be a relatively normal outcome of your present state of rehabilitation.

A woman who had once been a victim of the rare Guillain-Barre sydrome, a painful disease, perceived all reoccurring pains to be forebearers of the dreaded disease.

In contrast, a study done with soldiers wounded in battle in World War II found that the men needed less medication than civilians with similar wounds. The reason: The soldiers associated the pain with returning home.

Your characteristics. Some personal traits can contribute in determining your susceptibility to pain. These are low motivation, a poor self-image, a lack of pride in accomplishments, and a dependency on others. The element common to three of these factors is *diminished control.* With a poor self-image, a person becomes vulnerable because of his or her own perception of self, and vulnerable people do not often exercise control. The second factor, motivation, indicates passivity, which in turn indicates no control over time and energy. Finally, dependency on others is an abdication of control. All of these conditions serve to structure a person who is acted *upon* or *toward*, not one who asserts and acts.

A person with several of these traits is likely to perceive a pain stimulus as more severe than would a person who contends with distressing situations and possesses an attitude of normal, healthy aggression toward pain. This second individual will have an average or above average level of motivation, take pride in his or her own accomplishments, and be fairly independent.

Your perception of what the pain signifies. Your perception of what pain signifies is not completely separate from the other factors that have previously been discussed. However, for the purposes of clearly focusing on this influential element, it has been isolated.

A classic example of how this factor works has been cited by the present head of pain research at New York City's Memorial Sloan-Kettering Cancer Center. Dr. Houde relates the story of the young G.I. who was on a beachhead in the Pacific during World War II. As enemy fire continued in full force, one after another of his buddies were killed. Suddenly there was a hit nearby. He felt a screaming pain and a rush of blood down his leg. He yelled for help and was taken to a medical post where doctors discovered the location of the "wound" and the source of the "blood." His canteen had been hit and its contents emptied. Nothing more.

He went back into battle. Before long, he sustained another injury. This time he had a sharp pain in his head. He put his hand to his forehead and his fingers were covered with blood. On his second trip to the medical post, the doctor discovered a few fragments of metal on his face. They were removed with tweezers, he was bandaged and returned to combat.

At this point he was one of the few in his company who remained. This time a shell went off near him and he lost his leg. He felt nothing.

The soldier, in recounting his experience, said the most excruciating pain he felt was when his canteen was hit. When he had small wounds on his face, the pain was somewhat less. When he lost his leg—there was a complete absence of pain. Dr. Houde explains, "What pain signifies makes big difference in how it is perceived."

In the soldier's case, the first burst signified death. Everybody else was dying so, of course, he was too. He expected disaster. Contributing to his reaction were the emotional factors of stress, anxiety, and fear.

Another direct relationship between what pain signifies, its magnitude, and how it is perceived is illustrated by an experiment conducted with subjects who were to experience pain for research purposes. The subjects were directed to draw lots to determine if they would be paid nothing, $1, $2, $4, or $8. The experiment was conducted, and the degree to which the patients rated the pain's intensity corresponded to their payment. Those who were to receive $4 or $8 felt the most pain.

These two examples demonstrate the fact that the psychological component of pain is tremendously important. It is because of this fact that techniques that are psychologically oriented, such as hypnosis, can be employed with substantial success.

Treating Your Pain

The source of your pain will fall within one of the following categories: chronic pain; pain due to surgery; or pain due to injury, illness, or disease. As a victim of pain, you are joined by literally millions of others. Pain is the number one reason people seek medical attention, and pain killers are the most commonly and frequently used prescriptive drugs in our country.

Pain statistics are overwhelming. The pain of cancer is experienced by 800,000 Americans and 18 million throughout the world. There are 70 million with excruciating back pain; 36 million contend with the raging pain of arthritis; 20 million bear the blinding, nauseating pain of migraine headaches. If you include those with other health problems, such as gout, sciatica, and unknown causes, almost one-third of the people in the U.S. have chronic pain.

Your goal, regardless of the origin of your pain, is to reduce or eliminate it. Even though the causes of pain are many and varied, the results produced by hypnosis for the treatment of pain are much the same.

Chronic pain. Martha, a widow in her mid-50s, needed to return to the work force. She completed her training as a travel agent, purchased her own small agency, and began putting in 12 to 14 hour days. Before long, she was actively involved in the American Society of Travel Agents and was considered one of the most knowledgeable agents in her area. After eight years, Martha was the owner of three agency branches within her county. She was an authority on current travel trends and opportunities and was often consulted by others within the travel business.

Martha was a person driven to top her own accomplishments, and because she was largely responsible for the education of her three college-aged children, she had an added financial burden. All of this was compounded by a recurrent back pain. The harder Martha worked, the more pressure she was under, and the more driven she was to prove herself, the more persistent her pain. Martha's problem had a physiological origin, aggravated by tension and continual stress.

When Martha sought medical attention for her back, surgery was not presented as a viable option. She was given prescriptive drugs, which included pain killers and muscle relaxants. In addition, a series of exercises was recommended. But when Martha tried to treat her pain with drugs, her efficiency level dropped, her mental stamina decreased, and her personality suffered. She decided to try hypnotherapy.

The therapist taught Martha how to manage stress through the regular use of the *Relaxation Induction*. She used a *Specific Pain Control Induction* along with the *General Pain Control Induction*. Martha supplemented her inductions with positive imagery that reflected self-esteem. Within a few weeks, Martha's confidence had increased, and, as a result, her almost frantic drive was reduced. She learned to relax and control the muscles in her back. This reduced her pain and lessened its frequency. At present, she is more mobile, comfortable, and content. Just as important, while still a successful manager, Martha functions effectively without destroying her health in the process.

Pain due to surgery. Hypnosis can play an important role before, during, and after surgery. Using hypnotherapy prior to surgery can help you reduce anxiety and remove any negative feelings about anesthesia or the operation itself. During the surgery, hypnosis can serve as an aid to chemical anesthetic agents and in some cases, be used quite successfully as the only form of anesthesia.

Hypnosis can also make possible a positive postoperative period. You will feel more relaxed, experience less pain, and require less drugs. Side effects such as headaches, nausea, and vomiting, will be reduced or eliminated. You will be better able to participate in and accelerate your own healing process, and your sense of well-being and general morale will be heightened.

Ernie, a restaurant owner in Washington, D.C., had a history of horrendous dental experiences. Unfortunately, Ernie continued to need extensive dental work, including oral surgery, and he endured long periods of dread between treatments. His anxiety and discomfort were intensified by the fact that he perceived himself as a victim, not in control of anything once he was in the dental chair. The situation was further complicated by Ernie's poor reaction to Novocaine.

Ernie turned to hypnotherapy in a state of desperation. After interviewing him, the hypnotherapist devised a three-point program to (1) reduce Ernie's fear, (2) give him some control over the situation, and (3) directly control the pain. Ernie used the *Confrontation Induction* (in Chapter 7), which contained suggestions for reducing fear and gaining control over it. He also used the *General Pain Control Induction* and the *Induction for Surgery*. His positive imagery transported him to Hawaii to a beach in front of a condominium in Wailea. He was able to numb the area that the surgeon was working on, eliminate his great fear, and, most important for Ernie, gain control over the situation so that he no longer felt victimized. See Chapter 19 for more on surgery.

Pain due to injury, illness, or disease. There are no hard and fast lines between the treatment of one painful condition and the next. That is, the approach used for chronic pain can just as easily be incorporated into your treatment of a second degree burn.

In a typical induction for pain control due to injury, you are asked to use positive imagery and to watch the pain undergo a transformation from a symbol of discomfort (a red ball, blazing like the sun) to a symbol that is no longer threatening or harmful (a small ball that gradually changes to a cool blue and disappears). This is one way of effectively eliminating your painful sensations. The methods outlined for the other two origins of pain may work just as well. It is important to remember that necessary to any pain treatment is the need for relaxation and the reduction of anxiety.

In New Jersey, a young salesman named Larry was driving through the rain late one night. The visibility was exceptionally poor, and as Larry came around a sharp curve, he saw something in the road. When he veered to avoid the object, his car flipped over. Larry was unconscious behind the wheel. When he came to, he was trapped in his car and his abdomen was cut and bleeding. Larry had previously used hypnosis to reduce stress. Now he used it to stop his bleeding. He concentrated on the area that was bleeding, imagined shutting off a valve, and stopped the flow of blood. Help arrived and Larry was taken by ambulance for treatment, but his own contribution had lessened the potential danger of his situation.

Specific Objectives for Pain Control

To achieve a reduction or elimination of your pain, you will use three fundamental procedures:

1. You will transform, alter, or displace your pain.
2. You will directly address your pain and suggest that it decrease.
3. You will direct your attention away from your pain and experience the benefits of tranquil, peaceful imagery.

Programming for Results

The objectives above can be achieved in numerous and varied ways. The inductions designated for use in the treatment of pain are designed to help you feel, think, and behave in certain ways. As you use the inductions, you will be able to:

Experience deep relaxation to reduce stress and anxiety. The *Relaxation Induction,* the first component of your *Pain Control Induction,* suggests: "Just think about relaxing every muscle in your body, from the top of your head to the tips of your toes. Just feel any stressful thoughts rushing through your mind, feel them begin to wind down, wind down and relax. Notice how very comfortable your body feels, just drifting and floating, deeper, deeper . . . "

Transform your pain into a "visible" form. During the *General Pain Control Induction,* you imagine your pain to be a certain shape or form. This removes it from the category of the ambiguous, uncontrollable, and unreachable. The induction suggests, "Take the pain in your body and give it a shape and form, imagine your pain to be a tunnel that you can enter and exit . . . "

Own your pain and control it. The induction goes on to suggest that "the intensity of your pain increases for a few seconds." The purpose is to acknowledge and own your pain. Since it is yours, you can control it by intensifying it. Since you can intensify the pain, you can also eliminate it.

The induction continues with "as you walk through the tunnel, you can see the light ahead." Now you create an end to your pain by seeing the end of the tunnel. The induction suggests that "every step takes you away from the discomfort."

Visualize yourself as healed and strong. The *General Pain Control Induction* ends with the suggestion, "From now on each time you enter and exit the tunnel, you grow stronger and stronger, heal, and feel better and better." This suggestion programs your subconscious to heal faster and recover quickly.

Concentrate on the painful part of your body and heal it. The *Induction for Chronic Pain* suggests, "Imagine the inflamed sore area begin to reduce, cool, heal. Now feel the discomfort drain out of the [INSERT AFFLICTED BODILY AREA] and out of your body. Like cool water, flowing over your [INSERT AREA] and your body, like cool water flowing over your [INSERT AREA] and away . . . "

Numb the part of the body that is painful. You will numb your hand and transfer the numbness to the painful area of your body. (This is known as "glove anesthesia.") The *Induction for Surgery* suggests, "Your hand is now completely numb. Now place your hand on the part of the body [INSERT PART OF BODY, SUCH AS "your left knee"] that you want to numb. Now let the numbness from your hand drain into your [INSERT AFFLICTED PART OF THE BODY]. It becomes numb, like wood, heavy . . . "

Visualize and focus on positive images that direct your attention away from pain. The *Relaxation Induction* suggests, "You are in a [INSERT YOUR OWN SPECIAL, COMFORTING PLACE, SUCH AS THE FOREST, MOUNTAINS, OR A LAKE]. You are alone, and there is no one to disturb you. This is the most peaceful place in the world for you. Imagine yourself there and feel that sense of peace flow through you and sense of well being, and enjoy these positive feelings . . . "

Designing a Pain Control Induction

You will need to use two major inductions, each consisting of several components. The first major induction will be used when you begin to feel the onset of the specific pain related to your injury, illness, or surgery. The second induction can be used at any time, because it fosters feelings in you that will allow you to exercise control over pain in general.

To record the first induction, to be used when your pain is occurring, follow the directions for items 1, 2, and 4 below. To record the second induction for general use, follow the directions for items 1, 3, and 4.

1. Turn to Chapter 2 and use the *Going Down Induction.*

2. Find the specific pain control induction in this chapter that seems most appropriate for counteracting your pain stimulus. Select from the *Induction for Chronic Pain, Induction for Surgery,* or *Induction for Injury, Illness, and Disease.* Following the suggestions below, personalize your induction and record it immediately following the *Going Down Induction.* If Chapter 9 contains an induction directed at your specific health problem (such as cancer, colitis, cardiovascular disorders, migraine headaches, or muscle spasms), it can be added here to serve as reinforcement.

3. Immediately following the *Going Down Induction,* record the *General Pain Control Induction* in this chapter.

4. Close with the *Coming Up Induction* from Chapter 2.

These components should be recorded so that they flow together to make two total inductions. They will work together to meet your individual needs.

The specific pain control inductions are presented here as models. You should expand upon the theme of the suggestion you select; that is, it can serve as a *core*, around which you build a thoroughly effective posthypnotic induction. *What* you insert into this suggestion or add to it is determined by the particular source and characteristics of your pain. As you develop a personalized induction, remember to employ the key components of an effective suggestion, as explained in Chapter 2. Use *synonyms* for reinforcement, *paraphrase your suggestions, use connective words* to maintain a steady flow of language, and *designate time* ("in just a few moments," "now you will," and so on) when you need to signal the beginning or end of a particular behavior.

SPECIFIC PAIN CONTROL INDUCTIONS

Included here are three specific pain control inductions. Each was designed for use with a category of pain-producing problems. However, there is no binding rule about the illness, disease, injuries, or conditions for which any one of these can be used. If, for example, the *Induction for Chronic Pain* feels appropriate for you to use for your knee injury, don't feel that you must restrict yourself to the *Induction for Injury, Illness, and Disease*. The purpose of any induction is to meet the individual's needs. If one feels better for you than another, then use it. Results are more important than categories.

INDUCTION FOR CHRONIC PAIN

Focus your attention on the part of the body that causes you discomfort. [INSERT THE BODILY AREA, "your shoulder," "your jaw," ETC.] *Now recognize the pain and relax the muscles surrounding the area, relax the muscles all around that area, completely around the area. Feel these muscles relax and imagine the inflamed, sore area begin to reduce, cool, and heal. The inflamed, sore area will reduce, cool, heal and it will feel comfortable, very comfortable. Now feel the discomfort drain out of the* [INSERT BODILY AREA] *and right out of your body. Feel it drain, drain away, now just imagine a cool sensation, like cool water flowing over your* [INSERT BODILY AREA] *and away. The cool water flows over that area washing away discomfort, washing away discomfort, completely away, and now soothe and relax this area, soothe and relax this area, and now you can begin to feel relief, relaxation, and mobility again. Your* [INSERT BODILY AREA] *feels normal, healed, relaxed, and mobile. From now on your subconscious will keep your* [INSERT BODILY AREA] *relaxed and stress-free.*

INDUCTION FOR SURGERY

Focus your attention on one of your hands, direct all of your attention on that hand, and begin to imagine that hand becoming numb, recall a time your hand fell asleep and how wooden your hand felt. As you numb your hand, imagine a tingling begin in your fingertips and a warmth flow through your hand, soon all the feeling will drain out of your hand, soon all the feeling will drain out of your hand, all the feeling will drain away, and let this feeling be pleasant for you. Now let that hand feel numb, completely numb. Let all the feeling from your fingertips go, from your fingertips to your wrist go, let it drain out of your hand, let it drain out of your hand, let it drain out and imagine that hand feeling so numb, so numb, so very numb. You might begin to feel a warmth in the palm of that hand, a tingling in the fingertips, your hand feels heavy and your hand feels as if it were made of wood, let all of the feeling drain out and let the hand be very numb, so very numb, so very numb. As you concentrate on numbing that hand you can feel yourself slipping safely, gently, deeper, deeper, deeper into a level of total relaxation. Just let that feeling go, and let that hand relax. You can feel it tingle, so numb. Let it feel numb, let it feel numb, let it feel so numb now. Let the feeling go, releasing it, let that hand feel so very numb. It feels so very numb, as if it were wood. Your hand is now completely numb, feel it. Now place your numb hand on the part of the body [INSERT THE PART OF THE BODY, "your knee," "your jaw,"] *that you want to numb, place your hand on your* [INSERT BODY PART] *and now let the numbness drain out of your hand and into your* [INSERT BODY PART]. *Feel your* [INSERT BODY PART] *become numb, woodenlike, heavy, numb, numb, thick, as if it were made of wood. When all of the numbness has left your hand, place your hand back down into a comfortable position. You can keep your* [INSERT BODY PART] *numb for as long as you need to, as long as you need to, when you have completed just let go and feel the numbness drain away, drain away and your* [INSERT BODY PART] *returns to normal, when you no longer need it to be numb it returns to normal.*

INDUCTION FOR INJURY, ILLNESS, DISEASE

Focus your attention on your pain, now imagine your discomfort to be a large, red ball of energy, like the sun. Your discomfort is a large red ball. Now imagine and watch this bright red ball of energy become smaller and smaller, imagine the color of the ball beginning to lighten, beginning to change to a soft pink and reduce, reduce in size, as you watch the ball become smaller and smaller you will feel less and less discomfort. The ball grows smaller and you feel less and less discomfort, you begin to feel better and better, you feel better as you watch the ball become smaller, now watch the pale pink ball become tiny, tiny, smaller and smaller, watch the color change from faint pink to pale blue, it is now becoming a small blue dot, small blue dot, and now just watch it disappear and when it disappears you feel much, much better, you feel better, more comfortable, you feel better, more comfortable, very comfortable. You feel completely comfortable.

GENERAL PAIN CONTROL INDUCTION

Now take pain and give it a shape and a form, take pain and give it a shape and a form, make pain into a tunnel, a tunnel that you can enter and exit, now imagine yourself entering the tunnel. You are entering that tunnel and the intensity of your pain increases for a few seconds. As you begin to walk through the tunnel you can see the light ahead, every step now takes you away from the discomfort, the deeper into the tunnel you go, the less discomfort you feel, the light at the end of the tunnel grows larger and larger and you begin to feel better and better, every step reduces your discomfort, every step heals and strengthens your body, with every step you feel more comfortable, much more comfortable, very comfortable, and as you reach the light you feel relieved of any discomfort, you feel relaxed, stronger, comfortable, from now on each time you enter the tunnel pass through the tunnel, watch the light at the end of the tunnel grow larger, you will be comfortable and as you exit you will grow stronger and stronger, heal, and feel better and better. The tunnel is yours, you control it, and can enter it any time you like, any time at all, and passing through it will always make you feel better.

What to Expect and Following Up

If your pain is chronic, then a daily use of the *Relaxation Induction* will help prevent stress that weakens your body's defense against pain. If you have received the proper medical attention and use the inductions as suggested, you will find it possible to reduce or eliminate the occurrence of chronic pain. If you are to have surgery, you should use your induction every day for a few weeks prior to surgery, and, of course, on the day the surgery is to be performed. The *General Pain Control Induction* should be used in the postoperative period, until you no longer need it. If your pain is due to injury, illness, or disease, use your induction for specific pain control and, if appropriate, an additional induction component from Chapter 9, one that is directed at your specific health problem. You are the best judge of the frequency needed for your particular pain. However, it is recommended that you use the *General Pain Control Induction* for a week, then two or three times a week, until you notice a marked change. Then return to using the induction every day for a week. Finally, cut back as your pain decreases or is eliminated.

Special Considerations

Pain is a necessary and important condition within the body's system. Without it you would not know when you were injured or ill. Pain is the message that tells you when it is time to immobilize part of your body; it relays the message of illness so that you can seek medical help.

In order to understand what your pain is trying to tell you, you need to seek a professional diagnosis. Further, always consult a medical professional before making a decision about what kind of pain control technique to choose. If you have a condition that causes your muscles or joints to inflame and ache, you could worsen the condition by blocking the pain. You would not gain anything, for example, by taking your bursitis out onto the tennis court after numbing your shoulder.

A doctor should be able to give you an accurate diagnosis of your condition and may be able to refer you to physical therapy, acupuncture, or acupressure, recommend behavior modification, or, in some cases, psychotherapy.

In addition to discovering where and why the problem originated, try to determine what may be contributing to it—physical exertion, stress, anxiety, fear, or a poor self-image may be among the supporting factors.

11

Improving Self-Esteem and Motivation

"John's lucky," Art tells his wife. "Just plain lucky." That is the way he explains his co-worker's continued success in the face of his own continued failure.

Art was reading the morning paper at breakfast with his wife when he noticed another in-depth article on the economic slump of the real estate market. Art couldn't have agreed more, because over the last four months he had been receiving fewer calls from prospective clients and hadn't listed one piece of property.

As Art continued to read his paper, he thought that he might as well enjoy another cup of coffee. When he finally arrived at the office, it was ten o'clock—exactly one hour past his scheduled "floor time." He looked through his phone messages and found only one party interested in seeing a piece of property. He visited with his associates, looked through his other messages, and half-heartedly perused the multiple listing book. By then it was 11:30, and Art decided to wait until after lunch to return his one message. Perhaps a few more would come in and he could follow up all the leads in the afternoon. Art finally returned the call at 3:45 and received no answer. He waited until the next day, tried again, and reached his prospective client. The man was irritated and told Art that he had already contacted another agent and wouldn't need Art's services. Art damned the economy and went home for the rest of the day.

Art is currently missing days at the office. He has become depressed and finds it impossible to remember any success he ever had. Whenever he does make a business call, he is so unenthusiastic and unfocused that he dilutes his client's interest in seeing any properties. His finances are nearly depleted, and the worse things look, the less eager Art is to go to work.

John, another agent in Art's office, has plenty of prospective clients, is making money, and seems to have no problem finding financing for his clients. So, as you have already learned, Art believes John is "just plain lucky."

Art is self-defeating. He does not have confidence in himself to meet the challenge, and he sees himself as a victim of circumstances. He doesn't view the economic slump as an incentive to work harder. He is completely unmotivated.

John, on the other hand, sees himself as a winner and concentrates his abilities on turning the smallest opportunity into a sale.

The major difference in the two men is their image of themselves. John has a large dose of self-esteem; Art doesn't.

Self-esteem is one of the fundamental influences on nearly everything you do. When your self-esteem is low, almost all areas of your life—working, socializing, loving—are made more difficult. This chapter helps you to improve your self-esteem and then to program yourself for success by increasing your motivation. In the process, you will be given constructive procedures for creating a positive attitude and meeting your personal needs and goals.

Origins of Low Self-Esteem

Because a loss of self-esteem does not suddenly occur as a symptom at age 21 or 34 or 56, it is often not met head-on. You may be extremely critical of yourself. You may be afraid to attempt anything new. You may even excuse any success you have by saying, "I was just lucky," or "They made a mistake," or "Anybody could do that."

This kind of self-depreciation is not an accident; it does not materialize out of nowhere. It reflects a condition that is rooted in the past. *The major cause of poor self-esteem is past negative programming that is the product of judgmental parents.*

Because most parents are judgmental to some degree, it is necessary at this point to define the type of judgment that creates the problem. The parent who serves up a categorical classification at every turn, one who decides what you do is either *good* or *bad, right* or *wrong*, is one who fits this definition. You took 17 units at college and got four B's and one C, but you didn't get any A's, and so your grades are *bad*. When you were up to bat, you didn't get any hits, and even though you caught the fly ball that broke the other team's scoring streak, you were a *lousy* player. You answered the phone in your dad's office, took down the message, and exhibited good telephone skills, but you didn't ask if the call was to be returned at 3:00 P.M. California time, or New York time—so you are *incompetent*.

A parent who continually uses one-dimensional generalizations similar to the ones above is a *global labeler*. For example, let's say you are a junior high student who has been playing basketball with your friends since coming home from school. When you come in to dinner, your father asks if your homework is done and you answer no. Then your father says, "You are the laziest kid I've ever seen, just *lazy*." Your father could have said, "I'm worried about how you'll do in school when you don't put your homework ahead of being with your friends." Instead, you have been indicted, dismissed in a total way. In this case you are *lazy*. In other cases, you might be classified as *sloppy, clumsy, dumb, mean, cheap,* and so on.

Of course, the list of labels varies from person to person, and sometimes the labels that are the most condemning to you are those that seem to be most successfully buried and forgotten. But they are there, somewhere in your subconscious, contributing to the way you perceive yourself, influencing the degree to which you can exhibit self-esteem.

You inherit the "thinking style" of your judgmental parent. You acquire a critical inner voice that produces an internal fear. It may be a fear to try anything new, a fear to change, or even a fear to perform your daily activities. This latter fear is illustrated by the case of Sandra, a 29-year-old mother who worked as an English teacher in the local high school adult program. Her job necessitated driving at night on the freeways.

At a time when Sandra was experiencing a great deal of stress in her life, she began to be afraid of driving alone at night—even though she had done it for years. She had driven at night when she was a college student, as a night clerk at a railroad yard, and had already done so for three months on her present job. When she explained her fear of night driving to a friend, she heard herself say, "I feel *wrong,* somehow. I feel as if I'm doing something *bad*." Then Sandra was able to connect her feelings with the admonition she had received from her parents throughout her years in high school and junior college: "You'd better quit driving around in the dark alone, young lady. You're going to end up in some ditch with your throat slit. You're just out there asking for trouble."

In the past, Sandra had successfully buried that programming in order to get through college and meet her normal responsibilities. But when the other areas of her life became stressful, the old, inherited fear came back to shake her emotional stamina and reduce her self-confidence.

Fear of failure is an immobilizing emotional condition. It too is a product of past negative programming. You fear that you will not be able to accomplish something because you are not worthy of accomplishing it. Further, you tell yourself that if you *do* happen to succeed at one level, you will have to continue to succeed at higher levels. But each success will only make the inevitable failure harder to bear. You resolve this problem by telling yourself, "It's better to fail right now and get it over with." The anticipation of continued success would be much too hard to cope with. Thus, you can see that *fear of success* is actually the same as *fear of failure.* It is a condition that impedes personal progress.

Finally, your self-esteem may suffer from the way you perceive your physical self. This perception may cause you to miscalculate your overall potential. If, for example, you view your appearance as a negative factor, you will reflect that view in your behavior and actions, in the self-deprecating words you use, in your body language, and in the opinions you express (or fail to express). "I'll say the same thing Janet says because she's confident and popular." Or "I'm an outsider in this group, so these people won't have any interest in what I think.".

Instead of acknowledging your physical limitations and then mentally counteracting whatever may seem negative, you see your whole self as a negative. Consider the cases of Martin and Barbara.

Martin is overweight, but also affable and well-groomed. He has an unusual problem. Even though Martin does not overeat, he is not able to achieve any weight loss. His doctor has verified that Martin's weight problem seems to be a rare one that may be the result of a chemical imbalance. In any case, Martin feels trapped in his body and is terribly self-conscious. As a sociology professor, he never seems to feel at ease with his colleagues. He often makes excuses to avoid even small social contacts because he frequently thinks people do not really want him there. They are "just being polite" when they invite him. Martin would like to date, but he feels he is too unattractive to interest anyone. His value system has become distorted.

Barbara's poor perception of herself has to do with aging. She is a managing editor for a small publishing company in New York and is miserable in her job. At 48, she feels that any effort to try to better her position would be futile. If she leaves her present company, she will be unemployable. She actually inquires of a friend, "How can I go to a job interview with this wrinkled face?" She sees herself as a tired, middle-aged woman who, because she doesn't have her own company by now, hasn't "made it." Even though Barbara is a highly skilled, attractive, charming woman, she can't rally her own forces to go for an interview at a company that could provide her with a more positive working experience.

Both Martin and Barbara would benefit from a new approach.

Martin would have a more pleasant life if he said to himself, "I am a sensitive person who can offer warmth, intelligence, and loyalty. Lots of people would care for me if I just gave them a chance. They would see what I *am,* not how much I weigh."

Barbara would be able to better her position of employment if she could say to herself, "My skill and experience are what many companies are looking for. My 48 years of life have given me highly-developed abilities, expanded interests, effective communication skills, and organizational talents that have never failed me."

This positive approach is a product of *self-acceptance.* Martin and Barbara need to accept their physical selves so that they can shift their focus to their mental, social, and emotional characteristics and qualities.

These two cases illustrate a lack of self-acceptance in respect to appearance. Acceptance is equally necessary in relation to what you have *done* in your life. In examining this aspect of yourself, you need to say, "Whatever I *did,* my actions were the result of what I *was* at that point in my life." Your course of action was a product of your past history, your culture, your habits. It was the only self you had at that given moment. Any choice you make is a sum total of your awarenesses up to that time of choosing. This type of acceptance calls for you to accept what it means to be human.

When that acceptance is a factor in your psychological makeup and past negative programming can be eliminated, you can experience a certain degree of freedom in your daily life—the freedom from the tyranny of your own self-degradation.

Your New Program for Self-Esteem

Your major goal is to improve your self-esteem, not just today, tomorrow, or next week, but permanently. One way to accomplish this is by reprogramming your subconscious. This is done through the use of the hypnotic induction. Specifically, you will need to do the following:

- Rid yourself of past negative programming
- Improve your self-projection
- Increase your confidence and self-acceptance
- Change your perspective on your relationship
  to a given problem

Rid yourself of past negative programming. The parental judgments that labeled you *bad, wrong, clumsy,* or *dumb* need to be done away with. You need to see yourself positively, to banish the critic on your shoulder (or in your subconscious). The *Self-Esteem Induction* suggests, "See a blackboard with the uncomfortable labels that have been given to you in the past. And now take an eraser and erase those labels from the board, just erase each one, wipe it away, it has no meaning for you . . ."

Improve your self-projection. The *Self-Esteem Induction* suggests, "People see you as a good friend, worker, they see you as a good person. Just imagine yourself speaking to co-workers, bosses or employers. The words flow easily, people are interested in what you have to say, people notice you and regard you as a wonderful person. Just imagine projecting yourself in the most positive way, assertive, self-assured . . ."

Increase your confidence and self-acceptance. The induction suggests, "Imagine yourself standing tall, proud of who you are. Reflect on all of the positive aspects of yourself, your creativity, your intelligence, your talents. See yourself confident, very confident, you are certain of your abilities, your correctness, your talents, your appeal."

Change your perspective on your relationship to a given problem. You need to stop putting up roadblocks for yourself. You need to change the way you see problems and alter your response to them. For example, you no longer want to say, "I can't do it." "I'm not smart enough to understand it." "I don't have the energy." "I'm too old." "I'm not able to change." Instead, the induction suggests that you approach problems with these thoughts: "I can do it." "I have the energy." "I am just right for the job." "I can take charge." "I can solve this."

Using the Induction

Now that you have seen how your objectives for improved self-esteem can be met through the use of the induction, you are ready to tape your total induction. You will use the *Self-Esteem Induction* that follows, along with the *Going Down Induction* and *Coming Up Induction* from Chapter 2. The *Self-Esteem Induction* comes between those two parts. As you follow the directions below, make sure that each part flows into the next to constitute one continuous, smooth whole.

1. Turn to Chapter 2. Use the *Going Down Induction.*

2. Use the *Self-Esteem Induction* that follows.

3. Turn to Chapter 2 and use the *Coming Up Induction.*

SELF-ESTEEM INDUCTION

Now see a blackboard with the uncomfortable labels you have been given in the past, the labels that slowed you down and failed to reflect the wonderful, strong, and good qualities you have, and now see those labels on the board and now see each one and take an eraser and erase those labels from the board, just erase each one, wipe it away, it has no meaning for you, none at all and now the blackboard is blank and you write anything you want to write, and now you take the chalk and you write the words that describe yourself. You write confident . . . valuable . . . important . . . capable . . . and   skilled. And now you write other words to describe yourself. [PAUSE.] Look at those words. [PAUSE.] And now just begin to imagine yourself standing tall, proud of who you are. You are fine. The way you look and act and think are fine, they contribute to making you the wonderful person you are. Imagine yourself experiencing a new and healthy energy that helps you to accomplish all that you need to do. For a moment, just reflect on all of the positive aspects of yourself: your creativity, your intelligence, your talents. People see you as a good friend, a good worker, they see you as a good person. See yourself as a positive and worthwhile person. Just imagine yourself speaking to co-workers, bosses or employees. See yourself confident, very confident, you are certain of your abilities, very certain, you are certain of your correctness, your talents, your appeal, your conversation with others is easy, words flow easily, people are interested in what you have to say, people notice you and regard you as a wonderful person, just imagine projecting yourself in the most positive way, assertive and self-assured. You will approach problems with these thoughts: "I can do it," "I have the energy," "I am just right for the job," "I can take charge," "I can solve this." You are confident, capable, talented, and you have appeal. You are kind to yourself, you are kind to yourself, you no longer have time for negative thoughts or feelings, you fill your mind with positive ideas, productive goals, and you look at life as an adventure.

What to Expect and Following Up

Use your induction daily for about four weeks. Then, when you notice a significant change in your self-perception, self-esteem and confidence, use the induction whenever you feel the need for reinforcement.

Levels of Motivation

Once you have improved your self-esteem, you can work toward improved motivation. Notice that the phrase "improved motivation" assumes you are already motivated to some degree—and you are, in many ways. Psychologist Abraham Maslow has defined the areas in which people are motivated. The areas range from the physiological to the psychological, as follows:

LEVEL 1. *Physiological:* The need for food, drink, sleep, and sex.

LEVEL 2. *Safety:* The need to have protection, to be free of fear, and the need for structure and order.

LEVEL 3. *Belongingness and love:* The need to have social contact, friends, family, and intimacy.

LEVEL 4. *Esteem:* The need to have the esteem of others and to feel self-esteem; to be valued and important.

LEVEL 5. *Self-actualization:* The need to grow, to use one's potential.

You can see how you are already motivated in some areas of your life; that is, you have been motivated to accomplish level 1, and you have, no doubt, been motivated to secure your own personal safety, as specified in level 2. Level 3 seems to serve as a transition from these basic needs to those that are more complex. Level 4, *Esteem,* has been discussed in the first half of this chapter, so from this point forward the focus will be on level 5. This involves the type of motivation that extends into the areas of achievement and success.

To improve your motivation and, ultimately, your success, you need to rid yourself of any fear of failure, as discussed previously in relation to self-esteem. You also need to establish goals. Obviously, goals provide an incentive. But they also help you to (1) establish a sequence, an *order* for your progress, and (2) experience a sense of completion. Let's take a closer look at both of those functions.

Establishing a sequence. You probably know that your accomplishments tend to be dissipated when you work at many levels of complexity at once. That is, you can't engineer a design for a new computer program, work on the lecture you are giving to the university extension class, and settle the chaos that has developed in the programmer's department all at once. If these projects sound like candidates for a priorities list, that is because they are. After all, any structure is a set of priorities that make it possible for you to reach a certain level of growth or achievement.

You can see the same necessity for *order.* Let's say, for example, that you are a beginning potter. Your goal in the distant future is to teach private classes in ceramics in a nearby artists' community. It would be ludicrous for you to start planning for your one-woman show *before* you had put in your apprenticeship. Therefore, your order for reaching your goal could be designed as follows: (a) gain knowledge from reading, instruction, and apprenticeship; (b) work independently while seeking advice, opinions, and criticism from experts in the field; (c) establish contracts with gallery directors and owners; (d) submit slides of your work to be considered for shows; (e) show your work; (f) submit your application for teaching ceramic students in the nearby artists' community.

Experiencing the sense of completion. You need to feel that what you are doing and working toward will not go on indefinitely, that it has an *end*. Even life itself would feel fairly perplexing if we thought it were to go on forever. Working within limits or boundaries or time frames heightens the experience.

Now that you have reviewed the functions of goals, it is time for you to pinpoint your own personal goals.

Pinpointing Your Goals

In order to increase your motivation for success, you need to define for yourself exactly what you mean by success. You need to describe your goal. Here are a few examples of actual personal goals described by individuals in various situations and occupations.

Assistant treasurer in finance company: My goal is to locate a position for myself in a large finance corporation, one that would offer the possibility of promotion to treasurer and, within a reasonable length of time, promotion to senior vice-president.

Hypnotherapist: My goal is to concentrate my services in the areas of group lectures and presentations, principally at health-oriented and business seminars.

Graphic artist: My goal is to hire someone else to handle all my paste-up and layout work so I can concentrate on poster and package design.

Sales representative for clothing company: My goal is to learn all I can within this large company and then open my own boutique featuring clothes of my own design. Eventually, I will market my own line to other stores.

Doctoral student: My goal is to write my dissertation in six months, get my Ph.D., and achieve the status of full professor.

Notice how all the goals have a definite direction. A sense of movement is inherent in each one. The assistant treasurer is *moving out and up*, the hypnotherapist is *moving into a more concentrated, narrower area,* the graphic artist is *breaking away from and narrowing the field into two specific areas,* and the sales representative is also *moving from big to small* and then *spinning off* from her new center with her own creations. The doctoral student is being *upwardly mobile.*

Now take a look at your goal. Consider exactly what you hope to achieve. Then state it here:

My goal is to _____

_____

_____

_____

_____

Linking the Goal to the Reward

Along with any goal must come a reward in some form or another. Feelings of achievement and success are likely to come from any of the following kinds of reward:

- A sense of pride
- A sense of satisfaction
- Accomplishment on an intellectual, emotional, or social level
- Material gains
- The satisfaction of experiencing growth
- The development of your innate or learned skills and talents

Look back over this list. Ask yourself what type (or which types) of reward you are after. Your reward can be in any of the areas above, or it can be something entirely different. Your reward is as personal as your goal, and as long as it is meaningful to you, it is valid. To clarify for yourself the link between your goal and its reward, state your reward below:

My reward for [INSERT YOUR GOAL] will be _____

_____

_____

This statement and your goal statement will work together in your contract for success. Both statements will be used in your *Motivation for Success Induction.*

Of course, no success can be achieved or goal realized without a positive attitude. This point ties in directly with what you have already learned about positive programming and the major related factors—increased self-esteem and self-acceptance.

To get an idea of how concretely your attitude contributes to your motivation for success, you can check your responses to these questions:

1. Do I deserve praise?
2. Do I deserve to pursue a more specialized line of work?
3. Do I deserve a prestigious title?
4. Are my innate talents worth exploring and investing in?
5. Is increased happiness possible for me?
6. Am I the right material for management or administration?
7. Do I deserve a more comfortable life?
8. Do I deserve a higher income?
9. Am I the kind of person who can generate enthusiasm among others?
10. Can I maintain conditions that are to my own advantage?

In order to jump feet first into success, you need to be convinced that you are worth it. Both the *Self-Esteem Induction* and the *Motivation for Success Induction* will help you to see yourself as a worthwhile person, one who deserves to reach his or her goal.

Programming for Success

Now let's take a look at exactly how the *Motivation for Success Induction* will work to help you accomplish your three goals: (1) being motivated for success, (2) achieving success, and (3) enjoying success.

You need to have a positive outlook and attitude about yourself. Both a positive outlook and attitude are addressed at length in the *Self-Esteem Induction* which you will use as a component in your total induction. These factors are reinforced in the *Motivation for Success Induction,* which suggests, "Imagine that nothing holds you back from reaching your goals and becoming the successful person that you want to be. You are free of past burdens, you are confident, self-assured, you feel centered and strong . . . "

You need to program yourself to achieve specific goals. The *Motivation for Success Induction* suggests, "Imagine a goal or project you would like to accomplish. Your goal is [INSERT YOUR GOAL HERE]. See yourself put all other minor goals aside and focus on one goal or project. See yourself put energy into your work, see yourself complete the goal."

You need to assimilate success into your life and to enjoy it. The *Motivation for Success Induction* suggests, "You are happy, you are sensitive to others, you are helpful, your success is positive for all. You are comfortable in your success, you use your success in the most positive and worthwhile ways. Every choice you make and any path you take is absolutely right for now. See yourself successful, with many wonderful paths to choose and you know you can continue your success, can continue to make choices that enhance your life."

Taping the Induction

You will put your total induction together from several components. Each one should lead directly into the next in one continuous flow. Follow these steps as you tape your total induction:

1. Turn to Chapter 2 and use the *Going Down Induction*.

2. Use the *Self-Esteem Induction* from this chapter.

3. Use the *Motivation for Success Induction* in this chapter. Insert your own personal goal and reward where it is indicated within the body of the induction.

4. Turn to Chapter 2 and record the *Coming Up Induction*.

MOTIVATION FOR SUCCESS INDUCTION

Imagine that nothing holds you back from reaching your goal and becoming the successful person that you want to be. Imagine a perfect kind of day, a day that you awaken to and just know it's going to be the kind of day where everything is just right, everything just falls into place. Your feelings are good, you feel at peace, you feel content. You have been comfortable and protected within the boundaries that you yourself have created, you have been comfortable and safe, and now you choose to expand your comfortable space. Just imagine yourself pushing back the barricades, pushing back the barricades you created, and instead you are expanding your horizons, expand-

ing your goal, reaching forward higher and higher, feeling comfortable with your new goals, feeling comfortable with your expanded boundaries. You feel safe, secure, and pleased that you have the control and power within you to change, to change your limitations and be the successful person you want to be. Your feelings are good, you feel at peace, you feel content. Now just imagine taking this special day and placing it just a little bit in the future, a day or two, a week, a month, just a little in the future, imagine that you have resolved many conflicts, many problems, and they are now in the past. Imagine a smile on your face, you are at peace, content, you have found solutions to problems and you have resolved them. You are now free of past burdens, you are confident, self-assured, you feel centered and strong, now just imagine a goal or project that you would like to accomplish. Your goal is [INSERT YOUR GOAL HERE]. *See yourself put all other minor goals aside and just focus on one goal or project. See yourself put energy into your work, see yourself complete it. You see new opportunities, you see new challenges that are more exciting than the old ones. You see yourself with renewed energy, you are enthusiastic, you focus, concentrate, and new ideas develop from the old, new energy and positive feelings emerge, you are successful. You reach your goal.* [INSERT YOUR STATEMENT: "My reward for _____ will be _____."] *Imagine yourself worthy of all the good things life has to offer. Reaching your goal is very beneficial to you, and as you continue to reach the goals in your life, see them as positive events, positive for you, your family, friends, and people you work with. Imagine the goals in your life, see them as positive events, positive for you, your family, friends, and the people you work with. Imagine yourself putting energy into reaching your goals and becoming the successful person you deserve to be, reflect for a moment on other positive goals you have already reached, they were good for you and all those around you. Now see yourself become successful. You are happy, you are sensitive to others, you are helpful, and your success is positive for all. You are comfortable in your success, you use your success in the most positive and worthwhile ways. You deserve to be successful, see it, feel it, you are successful. Your mind is clear, you see yourself as the intelligent, creative and beautiful person that you are. You have many choices, many options, and whatever you choose to do, whatever direction you take, know it will be positive for you. Your success is a positive event for you and all those who touch your life. Every choice you make and any path you take is absolutely right for now. Now just see yourself clearly, in the near future with many positive directions and choices, and bring this image into the present, see yourself resolving problems, see yourself confident and successful with many wonderful and positive paths to choose, and you know you can continue your success, can continue to make choices that enhance your life.*

What to Expect and Following Up

Use the induction daily for about one month. When you notice significant improvements, you may want to reduce your use to weekly reinforcement sessions. For most people, this level of progress will be reached in approximately the second month. Thereafter, you can use hypnosis as a "maintenance system" whenever you need it.

At the beginning, you might like to keep a "success journal," a daily log that reflects success in any aspect of your life. You can note each time you make some small personal gain, each time you experience some achievement resulting from your increased self-esteem and motivation. For example, you can record each time someone asks your opinion or listens to you and takes your advice, each time you are praised in some way or singled out positively, or simply every time you feel more confident in your actions or appearance. It is only through small personal gains that big ones can result. Focus on what you accomplish and do not condemn yourself for the goals you have not accomplished.

Case Study

Cecilia, a 38-year-old nurse, had always been quiet and reserved. She believed that if she did her job well and provided expert care for her patients, she would automatically receive raises and promotions. Cecilia did not take into consideration hospital politics, difficulty with administrators, and working with a supervisor who seemed to know less about medicine than she did. The hospital was a jungle and Cecilia's job a daily battle, making it difficult to obtain the best medical care for her patients. The supervisor often overlooked Cecilia's requests.

Cecilia decided that she could contribute to better overall health care if she were in a supervisory role. She requested advancement, but her request went unrecognized for several weeks. She knew that she was qualified for the new supervisor's role, but she thought that perhaps she wasn't strong enough to effectively direct other people. She saw herself as a subordinate, rather than as a professional nurse who knew her job well. Cecilia had learned hypnosis to help relieve her patients of pain and stress. She decided that it might help her as well.

There were several areas in which Cecilia needed help. Specifically, she needed to: (1) improve her self-image and think of herself as the knowledgeable person that she was; (2) program a new image of herself as a confident person who knew what she was talking about and could communicate her knowledge in an assured, confident manner; and (3) use positive imagery to see herself as a supervisor, functioning effectively in that new position.

As Cecilia used the *Self-Esteem* and *Motivation Inductions,* she began to stand taller, to exude more pride in herself. She spoke in a kind but assertive manner that produced a positive response from the doctors she worked with. She again requested the supervisory job, stated her qualifications, explained her approach to the position, and emphasized her dedication. Despite competition from three other candidates, she was chosen for the job. Cecilia is now viewed as an effective supervisor who communicates well with co-workers and administrators.

Special Considerations

In addition to using the inductions, there are some other simple procedures to follow as you work toward improved self-esteem, motivation, and success.

1. Give yourself positive suggestions at bedtime.
2. Perceive problems as opportunities.
3. Exercise and eat nutritious food.
4. See yourself as healthy and capable.
5. Associate with friends who have a positive outlook.
6. Make contact with a mentor, a successful person in your field who can offer you advice and moral support.

Do a self-survey, and if you feel that you lack a positive attitude or motivation because you lack physical energy—if you are often very tired or depressed—you may need to examine, in detail, your health, nutrition, or psychological condition. Consider having a thorough physical examination by a qualified physician.

12

Improving Learning Experiences

Bill, a 47-year-old loan officer at a bank, has decided to change occupations. He is currently studying to become a stockbroker, and a position in a brokerage firm is open to him as soon as he gets his license.

After his first week of school, Bill plans to "study all day" Saturday. As soon as he finishes breakfast, he sits down in a comfortable chair in the family room and opens his book. After ten minutes, his son Peter wanders in and asks if he can switch on the Dolphin's game just to see what the score is. Within 15 seconds, both Peter and Bill are glued to the game.

At half time Bill's conscience gets the better of him, so he takes his book out to the patio, leaving the TV to his son. After reading a couple of pages, Bill's gaze strays over the yard, and he decides it needs to be watered. On his way back from turning on the sprinkler, he goes inside for a beer, then returns to his lawn chair. All in all, Bill spends about 40 minutes out of an entire Saturday actually studying.

There is nothing wrong with Bill's intelligence, but if his study habits don't change he won't have a chance passing the General Securities Exam. In this case, Bill's learning problems stem from not having selected *one* appropriate location to do his studying, not setting up a time frame in which to accomplish his task, and not having enough self-confidence to feel success-oriented.

All of these types of learning problems can be reduced or eliminated through the use of hypnotherapy.

Contributing Factors

There are almost as many theories about learning (and nonlearning) as there are people who want to learn. The range extends from Tolman's complex formulas to Plato's assertion that learning consists solely of discovering what we already know. In this chapter, we will deal with learning experiences that are based on study and examine clear-cut factors that can reduce or prevent their success.

Two major factors are *low self-esteem* and *lack of motivation,* both of which are covered extensively in the preceding chapter. Additional factors are:

- Poor study habits
- Poor memory
- Absence of reward
- Medicine and drugs
- Fear

To get an accurate picture of your learning problem, examine each contributing factor. Think about which ones may relate to your specific learning experience.

Poor study habits. Poor study habits involve both internal and external conditions. Internally, your sense of how to manage your time or how to bear down and concentrate may be poorly defined and difficult to put into action. This results in an unnecessary drain on your energy and emotions. For example, if you have an exam, a progress report, research to do for a lecture, a sales pitch—*any* act of learning that requires preparation and some semblance of organization—you can transform it into a traumatic, self-punishing experience by delaying it. If, instead, you did the task in small increments before your deadline, your task would be considerably easier.

Time management is not a complex, tedious process. It simply involves breaking your whole project into workable segments. You can do this with any block of material—the information to be learned for the bar exam, the research necessary for your annual report, the work of the three novelists that you need to study for your oral exam in twentieth century literature. Your learning module can be compared to an ice cube that you cannot easily ingest if swallowed whole; broken into pieces, it goes down easily.

The external factors of poor study habits have to do with the physical location of your study area and your *association* with it. A psychologist working with students who had poor study habits found that when the students followed the three rules below, their learning experience was markedly improved.

1. Designate one particular location for study and use that location consistently.
2. Eliminate any external distractors.
3. Leave the location as soon as you are no longer able to concentrate.

Hypnosis can help directly with the last two factors. Some external distractors will never be easy or even possible to eliminate. Your housemate's squawking parakeet or the stereo of Big Bad George down the hall are examples. (But you can learn to use hypnosis to block out sounds.)

Of course, if your external distractor is your baby, your spouse, or someone else close to you, then you need to settle on a study schedule that coincides with the times you are not involved in that person's routine. But you can't expect the people you live with to come and go as you please. You need to construct a cooperative plan of action that deprives neither party of his or her "rights."

The last rule, which deals with leaving your study area when your concentration has dissipated, can be regulated by specifying a time frame for your activity, as mentioned in *Guidelines for Effective Suggestions* in Chapter 3. This involves designating a starting and stopping time that corresponds to your normal attention span and then working within those limits. If, for example, you allow yourself condensed study time in the morning, you may stipulate in your posthypnotic suggestion that you begin at 8:30 and stop at 12:00 noon. Without a time limit, you could program yourself for exhaustion.

On the other hand, don't stay bound to your stopping time if you can no longer concentrate. When you can't focus your attention on your material, it is time to quit and *leave* the location. This practice will permit your association with the study area to remain a positive one. You will view it as a productive place where you can succeed at what you are doing.

Poor memory. A professor who was dining at the home of a colleague was "holding forth" after dinner. As the host and his wife grew weary listening, their guest continued to expound. Finally, the hosting professor said, "Well, it's getting late and I've an early class, so I guess I'll have to ask you to leave."

"Heavens," replied the absent-minded professor, "I thought we were at my house and I was about to ask *you* to leave."

A memory as poor as this professor's is rare. But if you find it a problem to retain and recall what you have studied, you are one of a large group of individuals who have some degree of difficulty with memorization.

We all have three types of memory, which seem to represent three separate "compartments" in our brains. The first of these, sensory memory, involves remembering the way something looks, smells, or feels. The second is motor-skill memory, which involves remembering how to perform a physical activity—skiing, riding a bike, diving, or dancing. The third type includes words, ideas, and concepts. It consists of everything you have ever thought, heard, or read.

The first two memory types are far more retentive than the type that deals with words, ideas, or concepts—which is, of course, the one which plays the most vital role in academic learning. To make this "compartment" of your memory function to its fullest, there are several simple procedures that can assist you in both retention and recall of material, regardless of the specific nature of the material.

1. *Self-testing.* As you read through, think through, or listen to the material, stop and ask yourself what the content is and recite the major points silently to yourself or aloud. If you can't recite them, go back to those key points and review them. The process of *immediate* review is more effective than rereading the entire assignment again.

2. *Periodic review.* An overall review at the end of the learning assignment should be done within a short time after the material has been studied or committed to memory. Reviewing *often* and *for short periods* of time will contribute to long-term memory of the material. A long, extended, torturous cramming session has less effectiveness in terms of successful retention.

3. *Break between tasks.* It has been proven that it is easier to retain two "blocks" of material if there is a break or rest between the two tasks than if the two learning blocks follow one upon the other. The assumption is that prior learning can interfere with new learning and that the mind needs time to absorb the prior material before it is presented with new information. You would not, for example, study for your psychology exam and then begin to memorize your lines for the community play.

4. *Use sleep as a "sealer."* At first glance, this directive looks like great news for those who want an excuse for putting their heads down on their law books and taking a snooze. The fact is, you will be more likely to retain information that is followed by a night's sleep than you will be to retain information you have committed to memory immediately before beginning your varied daily activities. Some theories also make a connection between dreaming and effective memory. It is thought that the dream acts as a straining device that filters out material that is unnecessary to the major objective.

In your lifetime you will be able to store billions of bits and pieces of information, some large, some small. For example, your private storage bank will hold more than 50,000 words. Some of these are easily obtainable, others may have to be searched for, but they are all available.

Facilitating any process of retention is the *meaningfulness* of the material to be learned. Studies have shown that people given lists of actual words to commit to memory had a higher degree of success than those who were assigned the task of memorizing an equal number of nonsense words. This supports the idea that you will be able to learn any type of material if you perceive it as meaningful in some way.

When presented with a learning task, the first thing you can do to make your job easier is to organize the material (mentally or on paper) into meaningful wholes. For example, if you were going to learn how to do something like carpentry, car repair, making stained glass, or tailoring, you could organize your information as follows: (1) tools or materials needed, (2) basic procedures to be learned, (3) results desired, and, optionally, (4) special tips for working effectively, efficiently, and quickly.

If you were to begin a crash course in basic conversational Spanish, you might organize what you need to know into "survival" skills having to do with basic salutations, eating, sleeping, restroom facilities, and directions. Later, you might go on to work on social amenities, expressions of opinion, and so on.

Memory can also be aided by organizing material into some sort of logical pattern. If you are studying a novel or a play for an English course, you would not focus on remembering every detail at the expense of the overall theme and plot. Instead, you would remember the broadest concept, the theme, then narrow your focus to the events that make up the plot, and go from there on to the other elements that emanate from the plot, such as characters, dialogue, setting, or symbolism.

Absence of reward. It is difficult to think of doing anything voluntarily without anticipating some kind of reward, however miniscule. You run three miles a day, and you look and feel better. You give a good performance or lecture, and you get applause. You contribute time and energy to a foster parents' program, and your day is fulfilled by the spontaneous smile of one small child.

In terms of reward, there is no difference between learning and these other activities. If it seems like nothing will be gained from learning, the task is made more difficult. If you can anticipate a reward, your resolve to learn is reinforced and strengthened. Therefore, if you do not already expect a set reward, you will benefit by constructing your own "pay off."

A teacher studying for her master's degree promised herself the reward of a backpacking trip after she successfully completed her thesis. You might reward a week of concentrated study with a long visit with a friend or a ticket to a play or concert. Rewards don't have to be elaborate in order to have enough power to draw you through the learning process. For example, you may need to take some time to identify a reward you had not realized existed—your own increased marketability, a heightened sense of pride, a skill transferable to another area, or the value of enhancing someone else's life.

You know what kind of rewards will work for you. Dole them out to yourself and don't cheat. If you don't study the proposal to be discussed at your board meeting, don't give yourself the day on the tennis courts you promised yourself.

Medicine and drugs. A lengthy list of prescriptive drugs can inhibit your ability to learn. The best ways to determine if medication is contributing to your specific learning problem are to discuss the question with the prescribing physician or ask your pharmacist to give you any available printed literature from the manufacturer of the prescription. This type of information is sometimes automatically dispensed with drugs such as birth control pills, estrogen, or pain killers.

Fear. Fear is an invisible but powerful force, which can, if it is extreme, seem to erase volumes of material that you thought you had successfully committed to memory. Fear has already been discussed in the chapter that deals with self-esteem and motivation. The fear which obstructs learning is a prime candidate for hypnosis. By learning to relax, experience feelings of confidence, and cue yourself to succeed, you can defuse a fearful situation. Your cue can be in the form of a word or phrase that gives you moral support. You may say to yourself "excellence is the only possibility" or simply "highest score." With such a suggestion in your subconscious, you are fortified for success.

Pinpointing the Inhibiting Factors

To expect optimum results in your learning experiences, you first need to deal with *self-esteem* and *motivation*. Without self-esteem, it will be exceedingly difficult to be highly motivated, and without strong motivation, the learning process suffers. Be sure that you have examined these conditions before you set out to improve your learning.

As you read through the list of factors that contribute to an unsuccessful learning experience, you were probably able to identify those that plague you when you study. Your first step in changing your learning situation will be to decide which of the factors—poor study habits, poor memory, absence of reward, or fear—has significantly affected your learning in the past. You will then state that factor and describe it briefly. For example, your statement and description could be similar to one of the following:

My studying is not successful because I have three locations for studying—in my kitchen, on the commuter train, and at my part-time job.

My in-service training is not successful because I know from past experience that my employer does not allow others to implement the techniques they learn. I'm not going to be able to get anything out of it.

My sales presentations are not successful because I can't remember what I had planned to say. I leave out important statistics and forget the descriptions of the new products.

After these negatives have been spelled out, the next step is to transform them into positive suggestions, such as these:

I will have one location for doing all of my studying. It will be at a table by the window on the third floor of the campus library.

I will recognize that my reward for my in-service training is the additional skill I am learning, and the experience which makes me a more "marketable" employee. When I finish in-service training, I will take that aerobics class that I wanted to take last fall.

I will remember my sales presentation because I will stop and recite the material at various intervals. I will review the entire presentation within a short period of time. I will practice it aloud at night before I am to give it, and then I'll sleep on it.

Now, on the lines at the left, state the factors affecting your learning experience and briefly describe the situation as was done in the preceding examples.

_____   _____

_____   _____

_____   _____

_____   _____

_____   _____

_____   _____

_____   _____

_____   _____

_____   _____

_____   _____

_____   _____

Next, on the right side above, write a positive suggestion for each factor. Note that the positive suggestions in the examples are highly individualized and made-to-order for positive programming. Later in this chapter, you will put each positive suggestion to work in your hypnotic induction.

Setting Up Your Plan

Now that you have pinpointed the factors that contribute to your particular learning problem and have created positive suggestions for changing that problem, you need to look at your overall objectives. These are the same for every person, regardless of the specific reasons for their learning difficulties. The objectives are:

1. To perceive the learning experience as an opportunity and to gain a positive attitude about it.
2. To change habits and procedures that are detrimental to the learning experience.
3. To improve confidence and self-esteem.

Reprogramming for Results

The inductions in this chapter are designed to help you think, feel, and behave in certain ways. They reprogram your subconscious by offering positive, constructive suggestions to accomplish those objectives listed above. Specifically, you will need to:

Approach learning with a positive attitude. A poor attitude toward learning can inhibit you from trying. If you feel that thorough learning is not really necessary and that you don't really need to apply yourself in order to succeed, then perhaps you are still the victim of some old, worthless programming that resides in your subconscious. If so, it needs to be banished. To change negative information from the past, the *General Learning Induction* suggests, "An athlete must learn how to move, he must learn the process of his sport before he can accomplish his feat. You are an athlete who is beginning the process of bettering your learning skills so that you may accomplish your goals. You can see yourself focusing, studying, concentrating daily, you are enthusiastic, eager to study because the results will be so positive for you . . ."

Reprogram your subconscious to replace all destructive and detrimental habits with new successful habits and procedures. Your subconscious seems to love habits and patterns. And you may have noticed that your subconscious is not very discriminating. It would just as soon commit your time and energy to daydreaming over a second cup of morning coffee as it would to striking out for the library bright and early. For this reason, there are four specific learning inductions, which work to counteract particular behavioral patterns. For example, the *Poor Study Habits Induction* suggests, "You will begin at [INSERT TIME] and you will stop at [INSERT TIME]. Within this block of time you will focus completely on the work at hand." In the *Fear of Exams Induction,* this suggestion is made: "Your stomach is relaxed, your chest, throat and breathing are relaxed, and now you begin your exam, you focus, you concentrate, your mind is clear and sharp, you recall quickly all of the correct information . . . "

Improve your confidence and self-esteem. If you feel that you are not worthy of being successful, are not a good learner, or you are not "smart enough," then you will be prevented from reaching your goal painlessly; that is, you might be able to reach it, but you will be engaged in a tiring, tortuous, uphill battle. You can achieve your goal more easily by fortifying your self-esteem and reconstructing your self-image. The *General Learning Induction* suggests, "You are confident of your abilities, you are intelligent and learn more quickly now because of all the learning you have accomplished in the past. You are talented. Just imagine how the athlete feels when he has played a perfect game, run the fastest race, or scored the most points. Imagine yourself as an accomplished athlete, successful, happy, and rewarded for your work, your consistency. You feel confident, good about yourself."

Designing Your Total Induction

Now you have an understanding about the way in which the inductions work. You are ready to put together a total induction that will meet your needs.

The induction you use will have four components, recorded in one, continuous flow. That is, each component leads directly into the next to constitute one effective whole. Keeping that in mind, follow this procedure:

1. Turn to Chapter 2. Use the *Going Down Induction.*

2. Select the specific learning induction that best meets the needs of your learning problem. You will select from the *Improved Study Habits Induction, Improved Memory Induction, Reward Induction,* and *Exams Without Fear Induction.* Into that specific learning induction, you will insert the positive suggestions you have written for yourself. Now record that

specific learning induction (including your positive suggestion) immediately following the *Going Down Induction*. As you record, repeat the key phrases within the specific learning induction and then repeat the whole induction a second time.

3. Next, record the *General Learning Induction* in this chapter.

4. Finally, turn to Chapter 2 and use the *Coming Up Induction*.

SPECIFIC LEARNING INDUCTIONS

Select the specific learning induction that best meets the needs of your learning problem.

IMPROVED STUDY HABITS INDUCTION

You are going to experience a completely successful study period, a completely successful study period, you will [INSERT YOUR POSITIVE SUGGESTION, CHANGING THE "I" TO "YOU." FOR EXAMPLE, "You will study at a table near the window on the third floor of the library."]. *Now just imagine yourself comfortable as you prepare to study. You arrange your materials, your papers, your books in front of you, you take a deep breath* [PAUSE] *and exhale* [PAUSE] *and relax, take another deep breath* [PAUSE] *and exhale* [PAUSE] *and relax, and you begin to focus on the work in front of you. You will begin at* [INSERT TIME] *and you will stop at* [INSERT TIME]. *Within this block of time, you will focus completely on the work at hand because you are enthusiastic and eager to absorb all of the information that you need. You concentrate completely, all of the normal sounds around you fade out as you find yourself absorbed in your studies, you feel calm, relaxed, and nothing disturbs your concentration, and you work at your peak, absorbing and retaining all of the information that you need. When the time is up, a signal from your subconscious will alert you, tell you that you have completed your work, and you take a deep breath and you are relaxed and have plenty of energy for other activities.* [REPEAT.]

IMPROVED MEMORY INDUCTION

Imagine yourself enjoying a day in your special place. Imagine yourself relaxing, smiling, playing, and feeling comfortable, feeling so comfortable, imagine for a moment that all your cares are far

away, imagine yourself lying down and stretching out. For the mo-
ment nothing is of any importance, nothing is of any consequence,
you have given yourself some time off and enjoy relaxing. As you
watch the day drift by, you feel so lazy, so relaxed, you notice a piece
of large, white paper drifting and bobbing on the breeze, and soon
the paper floats your way and as it drops near you, you can read
it and it has all the information that you need, all the information
that you have learned. You now remember all that you learned. You
will remember it all. [INSERT YOUR POSITIVE SUGGESTION, CHANGING THE "I"
TO "YOU." FOR EXAMPLE, "You will remember your sales presentation because you will stop and recite the material at various intervals when
you are studying."] *The information you learn will be clearly typed*
across a piece of white paper, and whenever you need to recall this
information, you will imagine that paper and know exactly what is
written on it. From now on whenever you need the information you
have studied, all the information you need will be written on that
large, white paper. It will all be there because you have learned it and
it is clear to you, and it is all there, all you need to know. [REPEAT.]

REWARD INDUCTION

Any time you learn anything you are adding to your own private
storehouse of knowledge. Whatever information you learn can be
stored and used when you need it. You may find that something you
learn today will become very helpful, very valuable tomorrow — next
week, next year, or even years beyond. What is important is that any
information you learn can be stored and used when you need it. When
you finish this learning task, when you finish [INSERT YOUR LEARNING
TASK, "your doctoral thesis," "your nurse's training," "your state board
exam"] *you will then reward yourself.* [INSERT YOUR POSITIVE SUGGESTION,
CHANGING THE "I" TO "YOU." FOR EXAMPLE, "You will spend a weekend in
the mountains."] *As you work, you can realize that you will have that*
reward, think about finishing your project completely and doing a
good job so you can get that reward. Think about finishing your proj-
ect, knowing you have done a good job, a complete job, a job that
qualifies you for a reward, and now think about working through
your task, remembering that everything you learn improves you as
a person, increases your knowledge, your worth. [REPEAT.]

EXAMS WITHOUT FEAR INDUCTION

Imagine yourself a few days or weeks before your exam, you have
studied, memorized, and retained all of the correct information that
you need. You are confident and you feel at ease, now become aware
of your stomach area, your throat, chest, if you are experiencing any
tightness or butterflies then relax this area, now once again, imagine
yourself before the exam, imagine now that you are prepared, you

have studied, and you are now ready, you feel relaxed, calm, at ease, now imagine yourself entering the examination room, you sit down, take a few deep breaths, and give yourself a cue, the cue word or phrase you have chosen is [INSERT THE WORD OR PHRASE THAT APPEALS TO YOU, SUCH AS "winner," "completely prepared," OR "error is impossible."], *and as you repeat your cue word or phrase quietly to yourself you can feel every muscle in your body relax, your knees are relaxed, your stomach is relaxed, your chest, throat, and breathing are relaxed, and now you begin your exam, you focus, you concentrate, your mind is clear and sharp, you recall quickly all of the correct information that you need, you recall easily, your body is relaxed, you feel at ease, you complete your exam methodically, confidently, thoroughly, in plenty of time, you feel great, you feel like a winner, and now just imagine the outcome of the exam to be positive, imagine yourself passing with excellence, with high grades, praise yourself* [PAUSE] *and now feel relieved, relaxed, and calm.* [REPEAT.]

GENERAL LEARNING INDUCTION

Begin to imagine yourself as a good student, a good learner, a fast learner, imagine yourself as an athlete who is about to go into training. An athlete must learn how to move, he must learn the process of his sport before he can accomplish his feat. You are an athlete who is beginning the process of bettering your learning skills so that you may accomplish your goals. Now just imagine yourself in a place that you have chosen as a study area. It is comfortable, you feel comfortable in this place. Imagine the time of day you have chosen for your study, and you begin to study and you focus on your work and as you focus on your work you become oblivious to any normal sounds around you, you begin to concentrate, absorb all of the information that you need, you retain all of the information that you have absorbed and you recall all of the information quickly and easily whenever you need it. It is just there when you need it and can be retrieved quickly and easily, you are confident of your abilities, you are intelligent and learn more quickly now because of all the learning you have accomplished in the past, you are talented and eager to reach your goal, you can see and imagine yourself focusing, studying, concentrating daily, you are enthusiastic, eager to study because the results will be so positive for you. Now just imagine that you have studied, absorbed all the information that you need and you feel confident, at ease; you are completely prepared and now imagine applying what you have learned and reaching your goal. See your goal in the most positive way, just imagine how the athlete feels when he has accomplished his goal, played a perfect game, run the fastest race, or scored the most points, just imagine yourself as an accomplished athlete, successful, happy, and rewarded for your work, your consistency paid off, you feel great, wonderful, confident, and good about yourself.

What to Expect and Following Up

You may begin by using the total induction daily before you begin to study. As your study habits become reprogrammed and automatic, you will need to use the induction less frequently. You should notice an improvement in your learning skills within the first week of application.

When you are preparing for an exam, be sure to use the induction well in advance of the exam and on the night preceding the exam.

Case Study

Todd, a University of San Francisco student in his late twenties, had always applied himself, and he had worked hard in college; yet, he graduated with grades that did not reflect his intelligence or the time he spent studying. His papers were of a high quality and he participated effectively in discussion, but when Todd had to take an exam, he froze. He decided that he could not remember the material, that if he did remember it he would probably remember it wrong, and that he probably would not interpret the questions correctly anyway. Todd convinced himself that every other student in the room knew more than he did. He stared at the back of the students' heads in front of him and wondered how everybody else could know something he didn't know.

Todd even had trouble passing his driver's exam because he was so anxious and afraid. Now he was preparing to take the M.B.A. exam. He had studied thoroughly and passed mock exams quite easily, but he was afraid that his brain activity would be immobilized when the real test came. Todd decided to use self-hypnosis to relax before and during the exam. To recall the correct information quickly and easily, he also used his own cue word that activated all of his posthypnotic suggestions. On the day of the exam, Todd walked into the examining room, gave himself his cue, relaxed throughout the exam, and did so well that nine months later he was sitting down to take his C.P.A. exam with confidence and success.

Special Considerations

Your learning problem will be greatly aided by studying the information in Chapter 11 on increasing self-esteem and motivation. As stressed previously, *learning* is very difficult without proper *motivation,* and motivation is closely linked to *self-esteem.* If you treat these three as equals, you will be more likely to experience optimum learning.

There is one fine point to remember as you reprogram your subconscious: Choose a time to stop studying, as well as a time to begin. If you choose only a starting time, your subconscious may not signal you to stop, and you may experience a flow of energy that leads you far beyond your intended time limit. This could burn you out very quickly.

Finally, there is one "luxury" you should consider having as you engage in any intense learning process. The luxury is a learning partner (or partners). This does not mean that you have to find someone with whom to study; it means that you could benefit from a learning associate. It will be helpful for you to interact with people who have the same goal, who are familiar with the same subject, or who value the goal you are working to achieve.

13

Improving Your Athletic Performance

In a cover story on the 1984 Olympics, *Time* magazine reported:

> The night before the finals in women's gymnastics last week, Mary
> Lou Retton, 16, lay in bed at the Olympic Village, conjuring. It was
> an established ritual for her, no different from the imaginings of
> a hundred other nights. "I see myself hitting all my routines, do-
> ing everything perfectly," says Retton. "I imagine all the moves and
> go through them with the image in my mind."

We know that gold-medal winner Retton executed an astonishing performance, notable not only for its mastery of skills involved, but for
its equally impressive grace, confidence, and charm. Retton was truly
a star.

As you participate in a sport, you may work very hard at training
your body. You push it, put it through its paces, and work for hours
to polish the finer points of your game or maneuver. However, all this
hard work may not train your *mind* to be athletic. One sports psychologist for a U.S. Olympic team says that 80 to 90 percent of an Olympic
athlete's performance is in the mind. This involves using your imagination, your thought processes, and your attitudes to provide incentive,

support, reinforcement, and refinement of your physical skills. It involves visualizing, just as Mary Lou Retton did.

Specifically, you can use visualization to do the following:

- Increase your agility
- Improve your coordination
- Improve your concentration
- Refine your technique
- Heighten your awareness of body position
- Eliminate inhibiting thoughts in regard to your performance
- Increase your capacity for enjoying the sport

In *Sports Psyching,* Thomas Tutko and Umberto Tosi discuss "Mental Rehearsal." They counsel the athlete to mentally rehearse the play, making it correct in all details so it will be a successful execution of the person's best effort.

Visualization, or mental rehearsal, is effective because of the fact that as you imagine an activity your neurons fire in exactly the same patterns they would follow if you were actually performing the activity. It is believed that these movements, along with contractions in your muscles, are responsible for improved neuromuscular coordination.

Along with the physical realization you gain by frequently executing your stroke, dive, shot, pass, or routine until you feel the sureness of it, you also realize an emotional affirmation. As you see the pictures in your mind, your subconscious is convinced that the desired feat is possible. When you experience the total success of your movement, you also feel the accompanying pleasure.

By stating your goal and then seeing it through, over and over again, you are affirming your own positive behavior. If you say, "I will be the fastest runner in the marathon," "I will score with every free throw," or "I will get my highest score in the play-off match on Saturday," your statements back you up and give you added power. If you can *think* it, *see* it, and *say* it—you can *do* it.

Take a minute or two now to decide on your immediate goal for your sports performance. Select the one area you really want to improve. Make sure you are *committed* to improving it. You can state your goal in the present or future tense, but it must be direct, clear, and positive. Write your goal here.

_____

_____

_____

You will use this goal later in the *Super Performance Induction* in this chapter.

Obstacles to Reaching Your Goal

Now let's take a look at the roadblocks that make it more difficult or impossible to reach your goal. Almost always, the obstacles are conditions that cause anxiety. Some of the most common are:

- Fear of failing
- Fear of being humiliated
- Fear of competition
- Feelings of intimidation

The mere thought of failing or looking foolish can trigger fear. The fear of being humiliated in front of a crowd or other players can cause you to tighten your muscles, change your breathing, and feel exceptionally tense or even ill. The fear of competition can have the same effects. You may experience a lack of concentration, an unfocused feeling—both mentally and physically. Your vision may blur, or you may get weak knees. Further, being intimidated by "better" players can lead to feelings of personal inadequacy and repressed anger. If you allow yourself to be intimidated, you may hold back from playing the best game you can play. You may not see yourself as being able to challenge such a fine opponent. As a simple illustration, assume that you learned to play tennis from a group of friends who are good players, some of them champions in local tournaments. As you improve your game, you do not realize that you are closing the gap between them and you. Instead, you still see yourself as a clumsy beginning player who has no skill and operates mainly by luck. Because you don't assert yourself and challenge the other players, they do not see you as an equal and continue to treat you as a less competent novice.

Eliminating the Obstacles

Regardless of the condition or circumstance that restricts you from performing at your peak, you can work to eliminate the obstacle through your hypnotic induction. Below, is a hypnotic suggestion that can help to reduce the barriers to athletic success.

HYPNOTIC SUGGESTION 1. *Imagine yourelf enjoying your sport, see yourself competing and enjoying it, enjoying it very much, and from now on whenever you feel afraid or intimidated know that these are negative feelings that restrict you from having a good time, from enjoying challenge, from exhibiting your skills. You*

take each one of the negative feelings and you place these feel-
ings in a box, just take each one and put it in a box, and now
put a lid on that box and place it in your closet. Now begin to
see yourself having fun, competing, doing your best, playing your
very best, you are secure and confident, you take your own
mistakes in stride, you are a champion, a real champion, and
just imagine for a moment any situation that may be stressful
for you, imagine any situation that may be distracting or make
you feel unimportant, and see yourself handle each situation
easily, effectively, assertively, and kindly. You simply refuse to
accept negative thoughts and feelings, they have nothing to do
with you, nothing at all, you handle situations easily, effectively,
assertively, and kindly. You imagine yourself playing your best
game, imagine yourself competing, winning, secure and confi-
dent, feeling that great rush of pleasure that comes from meeting
a challenge and doing it like a champion.

Working on Your Attitude

In addition to the conditions already discussed, other attitudinal problems can serve as impediments to your athletic performance. The most
common of these are:

- Inappropriate aggression
- Lack of confidence
- Lack of concentration
- Lack of assertiveness

The hypnotic suggestion which works on these particular problems
follows.

HYPNOTIC SUGGESTION 2. *Imagine yourself engaging in your sport,*
imagine yourself as you perform, imagine competing with
yourself or others, you are a good individual player as well as
a team player, you enjoy your sport, you enjoy exercising your
body and competing to test your strength and abilities, you enjoy
the social aspects of your sport, you enjoy your sport and your
attitude toward yourself and your opponent is positive, cheer-
ful, you are confident and strong, now just imagine yourself
begin, you ready yourself and you take a few deep breaths, and
you relax your entire body, you focus your attention on what you
are going to do, you focus your attention on your movements,
you concentrate, concentrate, you are able to keep your concen-
tration for as long as you want, you move easily and quickly,
you move easily and quickly, you are assertive, you are assertive
but not over-anxious, assertive but not over-anxious, not over-

anxious, you are steady and strong, steady and strong and you feel proud of yourself, proud of yourself, you behave like a champion, you are a champion, you learn from your mistakes, you are reasonable with yourself and your opponent, reasonable with yourself and your opponent, you are both human, you are reasonable, you see clearly the slight corrections that will allow improvements in your technique, you make those improvements, those improvements are made and you meet the challenge, you meet the challenge before you, you are ready for that challenge and you meet it, time after time, you just keep coming back with complete confidence in your skill, and you win, feel that win, feel how that win just moves through your whole body and makes you feel joyful, you are happy and joyful because you won, you have played a fine game, a fine game, and you now let each movement and each strategy be imprinted on your subconscious like a blueprint that can be recalled at each and every challenge, you are a winner, you are a champion, you feel like a champion through and through.

Ridding Yourself of Physical Symptoms

Still other problems are ones of a physical nature, such as:

- Shortness of breath
- Blurred vision
- Muscle fatigue
- Weak knees
- Tension
- "Butterflies"

The following hypnotic suggestion uses a cue to help relieve any physical conditions that occur before a game and threaten your performance.

HYPNOTIC SUGGESTION 3. *Imagine yourself before a game or competition. Imagine yourself relaxed, there is a smile on your face, you feel at ease, you are here to enjoy what you are doing, to enjoy what you are doing, enjoy your performance, you are here to compete and test your own strength and talents and to enjoy what you are doing, you know your sport well, you are skilled, talented, your performance is highly polished, you feel your entire body relax, take a deep breath [PAUSE] and exhale [PAUSE] and take a deep breath [PAUSE] and exhale [PAUSE], now feel your neck and shoulders loose and relaxed, feel your arms loose and relaxed, now feel your chest relax and breathe evenly, and now feel your stomach relax, just feel your stomach calm and relaxed, very calm and relaxed, and now feel your legs relax all the way down to your toes, just feel your entire body relax, and focus your attention on your toes and feel a comfortable, strong energy begin at your toes, enter the ends of your toes and flow upwards through your body, strengthening every muscle, strengthening every muscle, just strengthening every muscle, making every muscle strong, your muscles are filling with powerful, healthy energy. Imagine and feel it, you feel relaxed, and you feel steady, at ease, and strong, steady, at ease, in control and strong. Now lift one of your hands and gently tap your forehead, this is your special cue to bring about these positive feelings, to bring the energy up and through your whole body, to bring in that steady feeling, to bring in that feeling of ease, to put you in complete control, to put you in total, complete control, this special cue will always work for you in this way, it will always work for you. From now on whenever you need to relax, concentrate, and feel steady and strong, you can simply tap your forehead and feel these positive feelings flow through you, they will flow through you, quickly and immediately. Now put your hand back down to a comfortable position and feel the positive energy flow through you, your body feels wonderful, your body feels powerful and wonderful, and you feel completely healthy.*

Mental Snapshots

The short visualizations that follow can be used when you are in a fully conscious state, or inserted into the hypnotic induction, or both.

To use a mini-visualization during the day, you need only to focus your thoughts and see the image as it is described. You may sit down and close your eyes, or you may phase out when you are watching TV, reading, doing the dishes, taking a bath, or performing any automatic activity. If you can sit quietly and close your eyes, you will be more apt to run through your visualization again and again. As you do, try to imagine the sights, sounds, smells, and tactile feelings of the activity in which you are engaged. If you are running, feel the ground, the track, pavement, or asphalt beneath your feet. Focus your eyes ahead of you as you would in the actual race, breathe the outdoor air, hear the sounds you allow yourself to hear when you are actually running.

As you read the mini-visualizations below, you should consider altering the one for your sport so that it describes your athetic experience as vividly as possible. Use the short "snapshot" here as a kickoff for your own visualization. Rewrite it, including the sights, sounds, smells, and tactile feelings that bring your athletic performance to life.

TENNIS, RACQUET BALL, RACKET SPORTS. *Imagine your body in position, when you see the ball come, you move quickly into the right position, your racket is in the right position, and you hit the ball in the sweet spot of your racket; hit it with just the right amount of force, directing it out of reach of your opponent.*

GOLF. *Imagine your body position just as it should be, it feels completely perfect and natural, comfortable, now imagine a perfect swing, a perfect steady swing; you are in control and you execute your shot, making perfect contact with the ball. See the ball follow the exact course it should take, as you watch the ball it is as if you can make it go where it is supposed to go just by following it with your eyes, it's easy because your stroke was perfect.*

BASEBALL, SOFTBALL. *Imagine yourself up to bat, you feel calm, relaxed, the grip you have on your bat is natural, feels right, exactly right, you watch the pitch, you are completely focused, swing and connect with the ball, the ball shoots high, then higher, out of reach, you run the bases easily, effortlessly, you feel your joy carry you over home plate.*

JOGGING, SWIMMING, RUNNING, SKIING, BIKING. *You are enjoying your sport, you are breathing properly, your body is moving, stretching correctly, you are concentrating on your direction, your body and mind are in total harmony, you feel comfortable, relaxed, and energetic, you feel a strong energy flow through your body.*

Your Overall Objectives

You have reviewed some hypnotic suggestions designed to help alleviate certain problems, and you have read the mini-visualizations. Now it is time to consider what the total induction needs to do for you. Your overall objectives are:

1. To overcome fears and pressures.
2. To program yourself for a perfect game.
3. To program yourself to have a winning attitude.
4. To accomplish a specific goal for personal achievement.

To overcome fears and pressures. Your fears and the stress you place on yourself provide the greatest drawbacks to a good performance. How you react to pressure and changing conditions may determine whether or not you lose your concentration and ultimately lose the game or fail in your independent performance. The *Super Performance Induction* suggests, "For a moment imagine stressful situations that may arise, such as the weather, the actions of another player, or field conditions, and see yourself react to these negative conditions in a cool, undisturbed way, you are in control, you are unshakable, like a rock."

To program yourself for the perfect game. Your super performance starts (and continues and ends) in your head. If you think "I can't run the marathon," "I can't jog a mile," "I can't hit the ball with enough force," then you won't. Negative thoughts produce poorly executed moves, unrefined skills, and unfocused efforts. Begin by changing the negative picture in your mind to a positive one. The *Super Performance Induction* suggests, "Imagine yourself playing a perfect game, see yourself act and react, move perfectly, every muscle in harmony with your positive thoughts, see your strategy just as it should be, moving in, moving back, advancing, seeing every move, notice how you feel, you feel loose, relaxed, at ease, alert, and clear-minded, your vision is sharp, your reflexes are perfect, you feel great."

To program yourself to have a winning attitude. If you see yourself as an inferior player, you will not be able to fully use your skills. If you see yourself losing, you increase your chances of experiencing an actual loss. To experience complete confidence, you must have a winning self-image. The induction suggests, "You may reflect back to a time you played a perfect game and review all of the perfect moves you made, and all of the great strategy you used, this perfect game can be played again and again, you can play the perfect game."

To accomplish a specific goal for personal achievement. The goal you specified earlier will be incorporated into your induction. It will become part of your new self-image. You will be the person who accomplished that goal. For example, if your goal is "I will score with every free throw," you will insert that goal into the induction, changing the "I" to "you" ("You will score with every free throw.").

Taping the Total Induction

You will want to use a total induction that has the best possible positive effect on your athletic performance. To create an induction that meets your unique individual needs, follow each step below. By doing so, you can design a hypnotic induction with which you can feel completely comfortable.

1. Turn to Chapter 2 and use the *Going Down Induction*. This will allow you to achieve a completely relaxed state in which you will be open to further suggestion.

2. Review Hypnotic Suggestions 1, 2, and 3. Select the suggestion which best combats the specific condition or circumstance that

impedes your sports performance. You will insert this hypnotic suggestion into the *Super Performance Induction,* which follows. You may at this time decide to use the mini-visualization for your sport and to expand that visualization to meet your particular performance.

3. Record the *Super Performance Induction,* which follows. As you read the induction, you will find that it calls for you to insert (a) your Hypnotic Suggestion 1, 2, or 3, (b) your mini-visualization, and (c) your goal. Insert each of these in the place indicated.

4. Record the *Coming Up Induction* from Chapter 2.

SUPER PERFORMANCE INDUCTION

[INSERT HYPNOTIC SUGGESTION 3, IF APPROPRIATE FOR YOU.] *Imagine preparing yourself for the challenge* [CHALLENGING YOURSELF, AN OPPONENT, OR TEAM], *your equipment is good and is adjusted to your needs, you are prepared both physically and mentally, now just imagine for a moment stressful situations that may arise, such as the weather, the actions of another player or field conditions, and see yourself react to these conditions in a cool, undisturbed way.* [INSERT HYPNOTIC SUGGESTION 1, IF APPROPRIATE FOR YOU.] *You are in control and see obstacles as challenges, you are unshakable, like a rock, you are prepared and eager to begin.* [INSERT YOUR MINI-VISUALIZATION.] *Now review in your mind your entire game* [OR SPORT] *from start to finish, see it in slow motion.* [PAUSE.] *See it in as much detail as you can.* [INSERT HYPNOTIC SUGGESTION 2, IF APPROPRIATE FOR YOU.] *You played a perfect game, and now review all of the perfect moves you made.* [PAUSE.] *And review all the strategy you used.* [PAUSE.] *This perfect game, your perfect game, can be played again and again, imagine yourself reaching your goal.* [INSERT YOUR PERSONAL GOAL, CHANGING THE "I" TO "you."] *You have reached your goal, you have reached this goal and you can go on to other goals whenever you like. Now just imagine how you felt during your perfect game, imagine that confidence and ease, you were focused and strong; imagine yourself begin again, take a few deep breaths and in slow motion see every action, feel every move in the most positive way.* [PAUSE.] *See yourself act and react, move perfectly, every muscle in harmony with your thoughts, see your strategy, see yourself moving perfectly, see every perfect move, and now notice how you feel, you feel relaxed, at ease, strong, alert, and clear-minded, your vision is sharp, your reflexes are perfect, you feel great, and now see yourself conclude and win the challenge, you feel pleased with yourself, and every correct move, every play is imprinted into your subconscious so that you can repeat your perfect game over and over like a film, now go back and once again replay the sequence in your mind and this time at normal speed, imagine the sequence from start to finish.* [PAUSE.] *And see it in great detail, in great detail, imagine making all the right moves and playing a terrific game, playing a terrific game, the best game you ever played.*

What to Expect and Following Up

Begin to practice the total induction as far ahead of a competition as possible. If you have an event coming up six months from now, begin using hypnotherapy immediately. Use the induction on a daily basis for 20 to 25 minutes. If you are playing a sport on a regular basis, use the induction three to four times a week. If you have particular problems such as shortness of breath or weak knees, use the cue prior to each game or event. In a day or two you will begin to notice slight results; with continual use you should see a vast improvement in your athletic performance and mental attitude.

Special Considerations

Your athletic performance can be greatly improved by using the hypnotic induction only if other basic requirements have been met: (1) excellent physical conditioning, (2) well-balanced diet, (3) strong, well-designed equipment, (4) no use of drugs or alcohol and no excessive use of stimulants such as coffee, and (5) a receptive, healthy mental state.

14

Enhancing Creativity

A five-year-old artist summed up one aspect of the creative process this way: "Drawing is easy. You just think your thought and draw your think!"*

It sounds simple enough. But what happens when you don't have a *think*? There are times when any person who is actively involved in the creative process seems to find the imagination fading, the "flashes" of insight occurring with less frequency, or the ideas of no apparent value. Often, to complicate matters, fear takes over and slows the creative generator to a sluggish pace or seems to stop it altogether. *Seems* is an important word here, because it is highly unlikely that the creative process of an imaginative person ever stops. Creativity evolves from many sources, and it would be difficult if not impossible for it to stop entirely.

To understand how your creative level may drop, it is first necessary to examine the qualities and conditions that make possible the optimum creative experience. They are:

- Attentiveness
- Playfulness
- Anxiety and chaos
- Limitations
- Relaxation
- The trance state
- Receptivity
- Responsiveness
- Absorption

---

*From *Helping Young Children Learn*, by Evelyn Pitcher, Miriam Lasher, Sylvia Feinburg, and Linda Abrams Braun.

These do not occur in any rigid order, and many of them could, in fact, be operating simultaneously.

Attentiveness. "Originality," Woodrow Wilson asserted, is simply a fresh pair of eyes." While this statement is a bit too all-inclusive to be accurate, there is definitely value in fully engaging the senses, seeing things as if for the first time, and being aware of how things look, taste, feel, sound, and smell. The sensory memory of the creative person is generally quite strong. Scenes from childhood can be vividly recalled. Subtle distinctions of touch or taste are possible. What you notice, what you bring into closer focus—whether it be a tree, an insect, the way your friend moves her hands, the noises a child makes while playing—triggers in you a response. The response is not a duplicate of what you see, hear, taste, smell, or touch; it is a *reaction* to it and a *reinvention*.

When you perceive the world as new—every bit of it new—you will find fresh reactions within yourself. A 37-year-old woman writer, who had been mistakenly informed by her doctor that she had only six months to live, drove home from the doctor's office with her perception of herself and her life completely altered. Two hours before, she had been a normal person living on the earth. Now she was one of the dying. She began to experience highly-charged reactions to the slightest event in an otherwise ordinary day. Everything took on a new quality. Each shape, each subtle shade of color, each movement, became a gift. She wrote: "When I looked today at a sliced lemon, I saw, as if for the first time, the pale yellow, perfect miracle of it; in the afternoon I was struck by the unbelievable beauty of blue shirts flapping on the clothesline, waving abandonedly at freedom. Everything was fresh and had new meaning. And that evening the clouds thinned out, moving under the moon like steam, drawing a line across the black sky—as if, for me, they were underlining heaven."

The gift of your perception, which can recreate what you see, is both vital and compelling. Encourage it to be active, call it out, let it enrich your life.

Playfulness. "Play" is a loaded word, and when used in relation to adults the context is almost always negative. "What business," one may ask, "does an adult have *playing*?" In order to create, play must be an indispensable ingredient in your life; that is, often you will need to play with materials, concepts, perspectives, and to direct yourself away from those things that are real—to fantasize. Carl Jung has said, "Without playing with fantasy, no creative work has yet come into being."

Part of the reason children are so innately creative in their actions and their speech is that they engage frequently in fantasy. If you are a painter or sculptor, play with your materials. If you are a writer, play with dialogue, become your characters, assign Aunt Martha's speech habits to seven-year-old Jason. If you're a dancer, try dancing the way your name *feels,* the way a fire siren *looks* in the air, the way an orange *sounds.* State the experiment to yourself, then try it out.

Anxiety and chaos. As a creative individual, you will experience anxiety. Sometimes it may seem disruptive because it makes you feel empty, disjointed, unclear, without direction. Except for a small minority of artists with extreme psychological disorders, these feelings are both necessary and temporary.

In *The Creative Attitude,* Abraham Maslow stated, "If you try to be rational and controlled and orderly in the first stage of the process, you'll never get to it." The chaos has its place. The muddle you feel is an important condition that precedes the emergence of a new idea. You can compare this period to the way light is refracted in a prism. It comes in, is broken, and emerges in a dazzling new form that changes as you change your perspective of it.

Don't try to superimpose a sense of order on your thoughts and feelings in the gestation period. *Complete harmony during the initial stages of creativity produces nothing.* Your conscious mind and your subconscious need to grapple. You have no need to worry. The conflict is creating a valuable tension, and you won't go too far afield. The sculptor Henry Moore explains it this way: "But though the nonlogical, instinctive, subconscious part of the mind must play its part in [the sculptor's] work, he also has a conscious mind which is not inactive. The artist works with a concentration of his whole personality, and the conscious part resolves the conflicts, organizes memories, and prevents him from trying to walk in two directions at the same time."

Limitations. Your creativity benefits from having to function within limits. The poet Stanley Kunitz has said, "The hard, inescapable phenomenon to be faced is that we are living and dying at once. My commitment is to report that dialogue." This reflects working within limits on the grandest of all scales.

If you narrow down this perception, you see limits at all levels — and in all shapes and sizes. Can you imagine composing a concerto on a limitless piano keyboard, choreographing a dance that requires that you *never* put both feet on the floor at the same time, writing a book with words that have no clear-cut definitions?

Rollo May, in his *The Courage To Create,* states that "the creative act arises out of the struggle of human beings with and against that which limits them." One might argue that the more limitations one has, the more creative one must be — and the stronger one's creativity becomes. Nikos Kazantzakis put it beautifully when he said, "Man acquires the stature of the enemy with whom he wrestles."

Relaxation. Trying too hard, attempting to force a creative product, idea, or activity is deadly. There will come a time when your conscious work must stop and you experience a short interlude of relaxation. This is a crucial time. Studies have shown that during the crossover from the period of conscious work to the period of relaxation, the very idea the creative person has been hoping for and searching for emerges. The break away from concentrated effort allows creativity to breathe, surface, and bring you the "gift" needed to spark your work. It is important to understand that this product arises from the *alternation* of intense concentration and relaxation.

The trance state. Closely associated with relaxation is the trance state. You may remember how the various levels of the trance state were described in Chapter 1. You have your own light trance states which may occur while you are driving, jogging, doing dishes, taking a shower, or engaged in any automatic activity. Then your mind floats; your subconscious comes into play. Almost any creative person understands that, at these times, ideas come almost miraculously. Rollo May reports that Albert Einstein once inquired, "Why is it I get my best ideas in the morning while I'm shaving?" The answer, of course, is that he was at ease, engaged in a simple activity that didn't require any conscious effort, and his new thoughts were free to rise to the surface.

Most writers have had the experience of whole pieces of work coming to them as if there were a conduit reaching from the unknown to the brain. A poet reflected this experience when he asked, "How can I know what I mean until I see what I say?"

The first line of a poem, a bit of dialogue, the perfect title for your novel, maybe even a whole work, can come in the trance state, the *dream* state. Many exceptionally creative people have reported that ideas, words, and images often come when they are in a half-sleep state; that is, when they are falling asleep or beginning to awaken. Jean Cocteau described one such experience in *The Creative Process*. "The play that I am producing . . . is a visitation of this sort. I was sick and tired of writing, when one morning, after having slept poorly, I woke with a start and witnessed, as from a seat in a theater, three acts which brought to life an epoch and characters about which I had no documentary information and which I regarded moreover as forbidding . . . Long afterward I succeeded in writing the play and I divined the circumstances that must have served to incite me."

Receptivity. As explained previously, you cannot force creativity or *decide* that you are going to have an original thought or an insight. You can, however, acknowledge that the number of your new ideas is endless and be ready to receive one when it comes. This requires being alert to what is given to you, recognizing the breakthrough when it occurs. Such alertness is not a passive process, but is, instead, one which requires a high degree of awareness, a proclivity for recognition. Being open to the unknown and ready to acknowledge it when it crosses over into your consciousness is exciting. Emily Dickinson recognized this unidentified force behind her work when she said, "The unknown is the greatest need of the intellect."

Responsiveness. Once the "flash" from the unknown has been received, a response naturally occurs. The ideas flow and the judgment process begins. This means that you become selective. You ask yourself, "What do I keep and what do I throw away?" You trust your intuition, your past experience, your perception. If you have alternated conscious work on your creative problem with relaxation, your incubation period will have been a successful catalyst. It is time now to affiliate yourself with the mobility of creativity. You move ahead, you improve upon, you advance your original concept, you nurture, you incite. You are in charge.

Absorption. As you cruise along on the ecstasy that comes with the making of the truly new, the original, you will also become *absorbed.* Your self, in fact, may seem to diminish in light of the product you are creating. Your sense of reality may become distorted to some degree because you will be seeing everything else in relation to your creation. It may serve, for a time, as the center of your universe.

In *A Giacometti Portrait,* James Lord describes how Giacometti became so totally absorbed in his work that he did not distinguish his painting of James Lord from the actual flesh-and-blood Lord. Lord tells of the time Giacometti's foot bumped against the catch on the easel and the painting fell a couple of feet:

> "Oh, excuse me," he said. I laughed and observed that he'd excused himself as though he'd caused me to fall instead of the painting. "That's exactly what I did feel," he answered.

This state of complete immersion is perhaps the one that provides the most pleasure to the creative person. In this state you are removed from fear, and free (temporarily, at least) of the kind of self-criticism which can be so debilitating.

Delayed Creativity

Now you may be saying, "But how lucky Giacometti or Emily Dickinson or Jean Cocteau was!" You may be asking yourself why you can't have those same experiences. The answer is: You can.

Creative abilities (as well as certain mental processes) can be delayed, or temporarily diminished, but they are *there* and they will exhibit themselves. Their delay may be due to one or more of the following major deterrents (to which many other deterring factors are related): (1) fear, (2) self-criticism, and (3) excessive concentration that continues over a prolonged period without a break during the *formative* stage of your creative process.

Fear. The fear of the unknown extends into peoples' lives at every turn. And in each case it prevents progress. You've heard the all-too-familiar laments: "I can't quit my job because I don't know if I can get another one." "I can't get a divorce because I'll never be able to find anyone else and I don't want to be alone the rest of my life." "I can't go to a party because I might not know anyone there and would feel out of place." It surrounds us. Fear in the work place. Fear on the domestic scene. Fear in social situations.

Then there is the fear of the unknown and the fear of failure in the creative context. "What if I finish my novel and I can't sell it?" "What if no gallery will accept my work?" "What if my film is a flop?" There is no way to guarantee that success will occur, but it certainly won't occur if you don't take a chance. After Woody Allen had written and directed his first serious film, he summed up the chance he took by not sticking to comedy: "If you're not failing now and again, it's a sign you're playing it safe."

So you, as a creative person, can play it safe. You can immobilize yourself with negative "what ifs" and play it safe. Or you can mobilize yourself with positive "what ifs" (which are much more invigorating). "What if I discover a new technique that suits my purpose exactly?" "What if the critics review my book?" "What if the dance troupe choreographs to words, not music?"

Remember that all creative people fail now and then, because failure is inherent in the discovery process. As you work at any creative act, you engage in (1) trial, (2) repetition, (3) rejection, and (4) selection. That is, you first attempt something, you *try.* Then you repeat your efforts, discard what seems unacceptable for your purpose, and, finally, you choose. Now, if no one seems to appreciate the choice you make, your final product, that should not be of great concern. You have done what you set out to do, and you did it as well as you could. You need to see every creative process you engage in as a series of possibilities — and you are the one who is honored to preside over those possibilities.

Self-criticism. Of course, fear and self-criticism are closely related, but we usually think of fear as an inhibitor at the beginning of the creative act. Self-criticism often goes on a rampage once you have begun to engage in your creative process. It is as if you have a little critic perched on your shoulder who is saying, "What you are doing right now is not good enough, not original; it is silly, it is too bizarre, it cannot be understood — so why finish?"

This voice suggests, "You should be more cautious." "You should be restrained." "You should not be too emotional." "If you push too hard, you'll fall apart." "You have no right to be so pleased with yourself."

The result of all this self-criticism is a deflating of your concept, a dissipation of your energy, and a wounding of your spirit. If you allow your critical faculty to battle with your imagination and win, you consign yourself to frustration and, probably, a creative output that in no way reflects your potential.

You can get rid of this self-criticism by:

- Working in an environment where there will be no possibility of external forces substantiating any doubts you may have
- Suspending your own judgment and thinking only of executing your creative act
- Giving yourself permission to be awkward, dumb, silly, "crazy," emotional, or boring
- Being alive, open, expressive, powerful, uninhibited, daring, and curious

In respect to this last group of characteristics, Einstein summed it up when he said, "He to whom emotion is a stranger, who can no longer wonder, and stand in awe, is as good as dead."

Excessive concentration which continues over a prolonged period. Absorption and immersion are both necessary once you have launched your creative act. However, in the formative stages of an original act, when you are grappling with your creative problem (how to convey your characters' motivation, how to conceptualize your painting, how to formulate your proposal), you need to alternate conscious activity with short periods of relaxation. As explained previously, you can try too hard and block progress. Your seed, formula, visual image, pattern, refrain, must surface, emerge, or evolve. It cannot be squeezed out like toothpaste. Concentrate for a period, then loosen up and change the intensity of your activity.

Programming for Results

Now you know the qualities and conditions which make possible an optimum creative experience, and you are familiar with the three major causes of delayed creativity. With this information as a foundation, you may now use hypnosis as an aid to achieving these specific objectives.

1. Accept the necessity for unproductive periods during the formative stages of your creative process.
2. Dispel your fears and reduce your self-criticism.
3. Reinforce the productivity and pleasure of your creative process.

Each of these objectives will be accomplished through the use of the *Enhanced Creativity Induction.*

Accept the necessity for unproductive periods during the formative stages of your creative process. The induction suggests, "You are very intent on reaching your destination, you approach a crosswalk, the light changes from green to red, waiting for the green light you tell yourself the stoplight is only temporary, you take this opportunity to catch your breath and relax. You begin to notice how pleasant the day is, you begin to feel a new and healthy energy flow through your body."

Dispel your fears and reduce your self-criticism. The induction suggests, "You can feel a release from any doubts, fears, inhibitions, you can feel all of your creative restrictions fade away, you are free to create and invent, and now that you are free and feel at ease you are eager to find your creative energy."

Reinforce the productivity and pleasure of your creative process. You can program your subconscious to be receptive to your creative instincts. The induction suggests imagining a particular place that is conducive to creating: "Imagine any special place and make yourself comfortable, and now here in the most creative place, let your mind drift and say quietly to yourself, 'My new ideas can emerge, can surface, can evolve. This is a fine time for the new ideas to surface, a perfect time. I am ready to receive them, to welcome them, to use them.'"

Using the Induction

The *Enhanced Creativity Induction* is used with the *Relaxation Induction* in Chapter 2. You may remember that the *Relaxation Induction* was divided into two parts. The *Enhanced Creativity Induction* comes between those two parts. The three components should not be separated from one another as they are used or taped; instead, they should blend into one another in one continuous flow. Keeping that in mind, follow this procedure:

1. Turn to Chapter 2. Use the *Going Down Induction*.

2. Use the *Enhanced Creativity Induction*, which follows.

3. Turn to Chapter 2. Use the *Coming Up Induction*.

ENHANCED CREATIVITY INDUCTION

Imagine gathering all of the doubts that inhibit your creativity. Imagine just gathering them all and placing them in a sack. The sack now becomes a bundle of energy, you can use this energy, you can use this energy in a productive and positive way. You now choose to use this energy to accomplish goals, to create and invent. Now just imagine opening the sack and seeing a positive energy emerge. It is a brilliant color, a beautiful rainbow emerging, filling the room and enveloping your body. It is powerful, positive. You begin to see new directions, new ideas. You can feel this powerful force surge through your body. Your mind becomes clear, your mind is clear and focused, focused, you feel confident, sure of your talents and abilities, eager to set your new ideas into motion, and you control the energy in your life, you control the energy in your life, you are very successful at controlling the energy in your life, and now you can use this energy to fuel and encourage your creativity, to fuel your creativity, you can easily take these doubts, place them in a sack and change them into a brilliant rainbow of positive energy that you can use in the most positive and creative ways. Now just imagine yourself in a spectrum of colorful energy that surrounds and surges through your body. Now just imagine yourself walking down a busy street, full of energy, intent on reaching your destination soon, very intent on reaching your destination, you approach a crosswalk and the light changes from green to red, you wait for the green light, you tell yourself the stoplight is only temporary, you take this opportunity to catch your breath and relax, you take a few deep breaths and relax. You notice the neighborhood around you, there's a park across the street that is beautifully landscaped. You begin to notice how pleasant the day is, you begin to feel a new and healthy energy flow through your body. Now just reflect on your project and see it in the most positive way, visualize yourself approaching your project with a new and fresh energy, a new and fresh energy that is calming, soothing, and relaxing. The more calm you feel, the more enthusiastic and creative you become, and now before you know it the light has changed to green. You are free to go ahead, all restrictions have been lifted, all obstacles are gone, you are free to continue. You continue down the street and in just a few moments you will reach your destination, where some of your creative ideas and inventions have been waiting for you. It takes only a few moments, and the more relaxed you feel, the more calm you feel, the sooner you will arrive at your destination. Now imagine yourself reaching your destination. You are relaxed, you feel a new energy, you feel confident, you feel free. Imagine yourself approaching [INSERT YOUR OWN WORKPLACE, ROOM, OFFICE, OR STUDIO]. *This is your destination, this is your creative place, you have arrived, you feel excited, you are filled with new energy, your imagination is active, you approach your project, take a deep breath, close your eyes for a moment, open them and feel yourself begin, effortlessly, easily. You are absorbed, involved, there's a smile on your face, you are carrying out your own imaginative ideas, you are absorbed in what you are doing and all of your ideas are fresh, all of your ideas are fresh and new. Your body responds in total harmony with your thoughts and feelings. Visualize as clearly as you can these positive images.* [TAKE A FEW MOMENTS TO VISUALIZE THE SCENE BEFORE YOU CONTINUE.] *Let these positive feelings stay with you, they are easily recalled the next time you approach your project, and are easily recalled each and every time you need to create. Any time you like, these positive feelings will reappear, will fill you and be with you and you can continue on any creative journey you like where your ideas become clear, where all direction becomes so obvious, where all problems are easily solved. From now on, whenever you experience a block, just imagine it to be a red light that is signaling you to stop and take a rest for a few moments. Imagine the light changing from red to green signaling you to continue on your journey to creativity. You can imagine your block to be anything that you choose. A red light that changes or a wall that you can easily push and watch crumble before you, any image is perfectly fine. As you imagine your block disappearing, imagine yourself seeking a special place that will help you dream, invent, and master your skills. Imagine finding a magical path that leads into a beautiful forest, see yourself on this path, walking along, smelling the fresh aroma of pine and the clear invigorating air, now find a place where you can stop and rest. It may contain a cool and crystal clear waterfall. It may contain a massive boulder that you sit on while you let the warm sun soothe and relax your body. Or your special place may be a bed of fluffy down feathers that you can stretch out on and just drift. Imagine any special place and make yourself comfortable, and now here in the most creative part of the forest let your mind drift. Do not try to think. Just let your mind drift and say quietly to yourself, my new ideas can emerge, can surface, can evolve. This is a fine time for new ideas to surface, a perfect time, I am ready to receive them, to welcome them, to use them. As you drift you will see clearly, you will see new directions, new inventions, new ideas, and you can feel your imagination flowing, you feel an excited energy, and as you relax, your creative energy is released, you feel confident, at ease, secure in your talent. You can easily call upon your creative energy any time that you choose because all you need to do is to relax*

and recall your special place and feel your creativity, your imagina-
tion begin to flow, flow easily, flow easily, and now just continue to
drift, drift, continue to drift, continue to let your mind glide free, let
it drift, and in a few moments, upon completion of this induction,
you will feel free to create, to enjoy your creative talent, to invent,
shape, and form new and wonderful ideas.

What to Expect and Following Up

The induction should be practiced daily until you feel comfortable being
spontaneous, engaging in the creative process, and accepting your own
creative expressions. Once you feel that you are making progress, you
can reduce your use of the induction to one or two times a week; it
will then serve as reinforcement as you continue to pursue your creative
goals.

Case History

A group of 60 musicians, all guitarists, gathered for a weekend
workshop that was devoted to music composition and songwriting. The
workshop was held at a beautiful forest retreat with running streams
and lush, green meadows. All the participants came carrying their
guitars, pencils, and notebooks. The first morning of the seminar consisted of introductions, after which the students performed their com-
positions, in hope of obtaining feedback from the instructors as well
as from their peers. Many were too shy to perform; many who did venture onstage felt inhibited and performed poorly. The rest of the day
was filled with workshops, demonstrations, and exercises. That evening, an induction was given to the entire group to help them increase
their confidence and to enhance their creativity. It was suggested that
the next day, immediately after lunch, each person would feel a tremendous drive to create a piece of music. The members of the group were
instructed to imagine a favorite place in the retreat, to go there and
begin a song or musical composition. They were told that in this special
place their imaginations would be active and their creative energy high
and their new music would flow easily through their minds. They were
also told that they would be eager to share their music with the group.
    The next day, after lunch, the entire group eagerly dispersed into
the woods. Some went in pairs or groups; others went alone. A few
hours later, they all gathered together again. About half of the participants had written new music. The other half were now more eager
to share their music. Others who had been too shy now felt more comfortable performing. There was evidence of a tremendous improvement

for most members of the group. Doubts and self-criticism as well as fear seemed to have been significantly reduced.

Special Considerations

The creative person is susceptible to a few conditions that can be taxing and somewhat disturbing. Among these are (1) strong highs and lows, with the heights and depths being very pronounced, (2) exhaustion from absorption in a creative experience, (3) depression following a sustained period of productivity, and (4) health problems resulting from self-neglect or high anxiety levels. Hypnosis can work to reduce the magnitude of any of these problems, but cannot be expected to severely alter any creative person's basic characteristics, traits, and tendencies. Further, hypnosis cannot give anyone a talent he or she does not possess. But it *can* serve to release, enhance, support, and encourage a person's inherent natural ability.

15

Sleep

You've had a long hard day. The deadline for those reports that were due in three weeks was just moved up to yesterday. Little Billy's teacher called—Billy swore in class again. The Harpers, to whom you owe at least seven dinners, are arriving tomorrow night for an evening of fine food, fine food, and more fine food. You need a long and restful night's sleep. You lie in bed and close your eyes. But your mind is working overtime. A thought pops into your head and before it disappears another has taken its place. Time passes. You know that you need your rest, that you are not getting it, and you begin to fear that you won't sleep enough tonight to wake up refreshed or even coherent. As the fear rises, adrenaline begins to pulse throughout your system. You feel more and more awake and sleep eludes you for yet another night.

Since the deepening trance states of hypnosis represent a stage midway between alert consciousness and sleep, it is easy to see how the basic relaxation induction can smooth the transition from waking to rest. But hypnosis will be most effective if you first examine your specific sleep pattern and remove any external causes that may be contributing to sleeplessness. With a clear understanding of the ways that you may be stopping yourself from sleeping, you can design a powerful induction with long-lasting benefits.

Defining Your Sleeping Pattern

Your specific sleeping pattern may take one of several forms. You may lie awake for hours every night feeling miserable and anxious because you can't get to sleep. Then finally you sleep for a few hours. *Or* you may fall asleep immediately after you go to bed, but awaken in the middle of the night and stay awake until it's time for you to get up. *Or* you may sleep off and on for only a few minutes at a time. In each case you arise in the morning feeling exhausted because the amount or quality of sleep you had was inadequate. You feel the need for a more complete rest . . . rest that will make it possible for you to spend your waking hours productively without feeling fatigued.

Whatever your sleeping pattern may be, it has a particular cause. In order to learn how to fall asleep at bedtime you need to identify the cause of your sleeplessness. There are some serious deterrents to a good night's sleep. These may seem so obvious or simple that you think they don't require mentioning, but they do because hypnosis cannot be expected to overcome the following conditions:

You don't sleep because conditions that require medical attention or professional counseling have not been cleared up. These include alcohol or chemical dependency, chronic depression, chronic twitching or aching of your legs when you are in bed, and snoring accompanied by the need to gasp for air (Sleep Apnea). If you experience any of these conditions, it is necessary for you to eliminate the cause prior to using hypnosis.

You don't sleep at night because you consume too many stimulants (coffee, black tea, soft drinks with caffeine) during the day. You can't expect to include caffeine in large amounts in your daily diet and then slip into a state of total relaxation at night.

You don't sleep at night because you take a nap during the day. This throws off your sleeping/waking pattern and your body will not readily adjust to sleeping throughout the night.

You don't sleep at night because you participate in stimulating physical or mental activity just prior to going to bed. You can't run a couple of miles, work out, have a highly-charged conversation, or engage in a demanding mental exercise, and then plop into bed and easily doze off.

You don't sleep at night because you mentally associate your bed with activity. If your bed is the place where you field business calls, work on a report, write letters, watch TV, sew, grade papers, or balance your checkbook, your bed will be viewed as a center of activity. It should be seen as the center of relaxation. By associating your bed with sleep you are setting yourself up for a successful sleeping experience. (Sexual activity, of course, is the exception.)

If any of the above problems or situations apply to you, you need to take steps to fix them. This is a prerequisite to changing your sleeping pattern.

Examining Your Environment and Your Physical State

There are two areas in which helpful changes can be made prior to using the sleep induction. Any annoying element in your sleeping environment should be eliminated. And any tension in your body should be allowed to drain away into relaxation. By creating the optimum conditions conducive to sleep you establish an atmosphere in which the sleep induction will be most effective.

Your surrounding environment should invite total rest and relaxation. It should not be extreme in temperature. There should be a source of circulating air. It should be as quiet and as dark as possible, unless you find certain sounds (a tape of the ocean as it ebbs and flows) or a dim light comforting. Survey the location and identify anything which could disturb you in any way. Is there a clock that may chime or tick too loudly? Is there a phone that could ring? If you share your sleeping area with a partner, and if the partner is part of the problem (abnormally noisy or wiggly while he/she is sleeping) you may want to experiment with the induction in a separate sleeping area for a night or two.

Your physical state should be relaxed. In order to become aware of any tension in your body practice the following exercise after lying down in bed. Starting at one end of your body mentally focus your attention on each part (your feet, toes, calves, knees, upper legs, etc.). As you concentrate on the particular body part notice if any tension is present and if so release it. Pay special attention to the head area. Much tension is held in the jaw, brow, neck and shoulders. See if you can notice any area which aches from being held tight during the day. If so, focus your attention there and concentrate on relaxing that area.

Typical Bedtime Monologues

When you go to bed your mind must also begin to relax, to let go of the problems and events of the day. Consider now what your mind does when you try to sleep. Think about the kinds of thoughts that go through your mind when you are in bed. Here are three types of monologues that may sound familiar to you.

The Clock Watcher: "Oh no, it's one thirty in the morning. I've been in bed since eleven and I still can't get to sleep. What can I do? I won't be able to work tomorrow. I'll look worn out and drained. I'll feel terrible. Oh no, now it's almost two o'clock. Even if I get to sleep in five minutes I'll only be able to sleep four hours. I can't get by on only four hours sleep."

The Doomsayer: "I can't sleep and I'm completely miserable. Everything is messed up lately anyway. I can't seem to make anything work out. Not even getting to sleep. Life is just one negative experience after another. Now insomnia is *another* punishment I have to endure."

The Fixer: "I have to figure a way out of this one or I am going to be in deep trouble . . . What if I try to . . . I'll say this to him and this is what he'll say back . . . Oh, there's no way out and all I can do is go around in circles. What if I . . . ."

Think about the category or categories in which you see yourself. Many people find themselves in all three categories. If you do, this simply means that you are keeping yourself awake using three different methods, all of which are enormously successful. Take a moment here to identify the category into which your bedtime thought processes fit.

Reprogramming for Results

The inductions in this chapter are designed to help you re-pattern your mental activity so that your mind is calm and peaceful before you go to sleep. When it's time for you to rest, your body and mind will be at ease and allow you to gently drift off to sleep. The following positive suggestions can replace your usual bedtime monologue.

Give yourself permission to rest while awake. If you are a *clock watcher* this means you work yourself into a highly anxious state over the fact that more and more time keeps ticking by and you are not yet asleep. You need, therefore, to direct your thoughts away from the passage of time; you need to stop looking at the clock. Instead you'll tell yourself that you are resting and resting is the first step to sleep. You actually say to yourself, "Time is unimportant and I am resting as my mind floats. Resting puts my mind and body at ease." Look at this two-sentence statement. This is the new thought that will help you develop new behavior. You are no longer going to be a *clock watcher.* From now on this label no longer describes you.

Replace the negative with a positive. If you identified yourself as a *doomsayer,* you view your lack of sleep as just another negative life experience beyond your control. Instead, you need to remind yourself of the good things that have come your way during the day. You may have received positive feedback at work. You may have been praised for something you said or did. You may have received a compliment about how you looked or an invitation from someone who obviously seeks out and values your company. Focus away from those things which cause you to feel helpless, like a victim. You aren't. Instead of doomsaying, practice saying the following affirmation: "Several good things have happened to me today. More positive things will happen tomorrow." This is the new thought that will help establish your new behavior. You are not a *doomsayer* any longer. This label no longer describes you.

Relate night time to sleep time. If you identified with the fixer you need to put away your problems, whether they are real or imaginary. Table them until you are required to deal with them during the natural course of a day's events. If you are a *fixer* repeat the following to yourself: "I will put away my problems at night. I will deal with them at a better time. " Again, this is the new thought that will help you with your new behavior. It is your positive suggestion. From now on you will not be a nighttime *fixer*.

Now pick the positive suggestions that apply to you from the above categories and write them down. This is the contract for your new behavior. In the hypnotic induction you will see this contract. You will incorporate these positive suggestions into your subconscious. You will no longer focus on time. You will not tell yourself how negative life is. You will not solve or create problems. You will not view yourself as insomnia's victim. You have written down your new behavior and will incorporate it both consciously and subconsciously.

The Total Induction

Since your objective is to remain asleep throughout the night, you will not need to use the *Coming Up Induction*. In the *Sleep Induction* you'll visualize your contract with the positive suggestions in writing. By reviewing these statements in a trance you reprogram your subconscious to replace old mental patterns with new positive, relaxing, mental activity. During the *Sleep Induction* your subconscious will accept three suggestions: that you will go to sleep quickly, that you will not awaken during the night unless you need to, and that you will have a restful sleep and awaken in the morning feeling refreshed.

1. Turn to Chapter 2 and record the *Going Down Induction*.

2. Use the *Sleep Induction* that follows.

SLEEP INDUCTION

And now just linger in your special place. There's no place to go, nothing to do. Just rest, just let yourself drift and float, drift and float into a sound and restful sleep. And as you drift deeper and deeper visualize your contract. See what you have written there. See those positive statements, ideas, and goals. See what you have written and know that it is true. Your new positive thoughts are true. You have released negative thoughts and feelings. You have released stress and tension from your mind, body, and thoughts. Each new positive statement becomes stronger and stronger as you continue to drift deeper and deeper into relaxation. Just let yourself drift deeper and deeper into sleep. Just let those positive statements float in your mind as you drift into a sound and restful sleep. And now become aware of how comfortable you feel, so relaxed, your head and shoulders are in just the right position, your back is supported, and you are becoming less and less aware of all the normal sounds of your surroundings, and as you drift deeper and deeper you may experience a negative thought or worry trying to surface in your mind, trying to disrupt your slumber, trying to disrupt your rest. Simply take that thought, sweep it up as you would sweep up crumbs from the floor, and place that thought or worry into the box. The box has a nice tight lid. Put the lid on the box and place the box on the top shelf of your closet. You can go back to that box at another time, a time that is more appropriate, a time that will not interfere with your sleep. So as these unwanted thoughts appear, sweep them up and place them in the box, put a lid on the box and place it on the top shelf of your closet and let them go. Let them go and continue to drift deeper and deeper into sleep. Shift your thoughts back to your positive thoughts and positive statements. Just let these thoughts flow through your mind, thoughts such as "I am a worthwhile person." [PAUSE] *"I have accomplished many good things."* [PAUSE] *"I have reached positive goals."* [PAUSE] *Just let your own positive ideas flow through your mind. Let them flow and drift, becoming stronger and stronger as you drift deeper and deeper into sleep. You may begin to see them slowly fade, slowly fade as you become even more relaxed, more sleepy, more drowsy, more relaxed. Just imagine yourself in your peaceful and special place, smiling, feeling so good, so comfortable, so relaxed.* [PAUSE] *And from your special place you can easily drift into a sound and restful sleep, a sound and restful sleep, undisturbed in a sound and restful sleep. You sleep throughout the night in a sound and restful sleep. If you should awaken you simply imagine your special place once again, and drift easily back into a sound and restful sleep, a sound and restful sleep. Your breathing becomes so relaxed, your thoughts wind down, wind down, wind down and relax. You drift and float into a sound and restful sleep, undisturbed throughout the night. You will awaken at your designated time feeling rested and refreshed. Now there's nothing to do, nothing to think about, nothing to do but enjoy your special place, your special place that is so peaceful for you, so relaxing. Just imagine how it feels to relax in your special place. You may become aware of how clean and fresh your special place smells, or you may become aware of the different sounds of your special place, such as birds singing in the background, or water cascading over river rocks in a stream. Or you may become aware of how warm the sun feels as you lounge in a hammock, or how cool the breeze feels from the ocean air. Or you may experience something else that is unique and wonderful in your special place. just experience it, drift and float, all thoughts just fading, drifting into a sound and restful sleep. Just drift into a comfortable, cozy, restful sleep, your body feeling heavy and relaxed as you sink into your bed, so relaxed, just drifting into sleep* [PAUSE], *sleep* [PAUSE], *sleep* [PAUSE SOFTLY REPEAT SLEEP 3 MORE TIMES], *sleep . . . sleep . . . sleep . . .*

16

Anxiety and Panic

This chapter and induction is adapted from an audiotape of the same name written by Matthew McKay.

It's a warm, spring day. The smell of honeysuckle permeates the air. You are walking down a wide, tree-lined street to go to a baby shower for your best friend, Anna. As you walk, a cloud passes over the sun. The air becomes slightly chilled. A sudden gust of wind rustles the tree branches, and for a moment the atmosphere seems darker, colder, almost menacing. As you continue, you notice the sound of footsteps behind you and, for no apparent reason, you wonder whether these steps are purposely keeping pace with yours. Although you are still in the same friendly neighborhood on the same springlike day, a thought crosses your mind: "Maybe I'm about to be mugged." As the steps come closer your heart starts to race, your cheeks become flushed. You suddenly feel very dizzy, as though you will faint where you stand. At the point when you become certain you can't tolerate the fear, the sound of the footsteps turns off onto a side street. You look around and see the mail carrier rounding the corner of the Nugent's house.

Contrary to popular belief, anxiety does not arise directly out of dangerous or painful situations. Anxiety actually arises out of your thoughts. In a given situation, it's the thought of potential danger, not the actual danger, that produces the symptoms of anxiety.

The ABCs of Anxiety

The process described above is often called the ABC model of anxiety—the situation, A, gives rise to the thought, B, which in turn causes the anxiety, C. This ABC sequence can escalate by virtue of a feedback loop. This happens when the feeling of the anxiety itself becomes the stimulus for a further catastrophic thought. You make a second prediction to yourself, such as "I feel scared. This is really dangerous." The new catastrophic thought makes you feel even more anxious, which prompts more thoughts about the danger, and so on.

This type of emotional escalation is particularly difficult to stop when you're in a situation that you can't avoid: at a party you can't leave, for example. Or at work, where you fear your boss's anger, but you can't go home. Or when you feel an unusual pain or sensation in your body. In these types of situations you feel as though you are not in control and that an added danger exists: the situation might overwhelm you.

Your anxiety can be managed as long as your thoughts about difficult situations are realistic and accurate. But if you overestimate the danger and continually predict disaster, your anxiety will increase dramatically. If you tell yourself "I'm going to be attacked" when you are standing next to a policeman on a busy downtown street, that's not a rational belief. You're predicting danger where almost none exists. The same process occurs if you do a good job at work, but constantly say to yourself, "What if the boss doesn't like my work? What if he fires me? I'll never get another job."

Panic Mechanics

Panic escalation usually exhibits four distinct phases.

1. **You make unrealistic self-statements that keep you in a constant state of alarm.** Your body tenses in the fight-or-flight reaction: your heart beats faster, you feel short of breath, you have butterflies in your stomach, and so on. This chronic state of arousal makes you "sensitized" to any hint of possible danger. Sensitization means that your nerves are set on a hair trigger. The least reversal, unpleasant surprise, or minor conflict can set off a siege of panic.
2. **You begin to fear fear itself.** As your body becomes more sensitized, you begin to anticipate panic attacks. You try to avoid them at all costs. Now you have a new fear. You not only fear the violence or the boss's criticism, you also dread the symptoms that fear causes in your body.

3. **You reject your own feelings as your fear of fear escalates.** You hate experiencing the symptoms of your fear: the pounding heart, the dizziness, the shortness of breath, the trembling legs, the lump in your throat, the hot or cold flashes, and the confusion you feel in your mind. You resist and fight against anything unusual happening in your body. You become hypervigilant for symptoms of an approaching panic. You come to fear any emotion or experience that triggers physical sensations that remind you of panic. Even feeling excited, exercising, or contracting innocuous illnesses such as the flu seems dangerous because the symptoms remind you of the feeling of panic.

4. **You avoid, ultimately, any situation, person, or thing that evokes feelings of arousal or anxiety.** What started as nervousness when walking empty streets becomes avoidance of going anywhere alone. What started as anxious thoughts when talking to the boss becomes avoidance of work altogether. What started as painful shyness at parties becomes avoidance of every social contact.

Fortunately there is a way to cope with this nightmare of anxiety and panic. The hypnotic inductions in this chapter can help you relax, accept the alarming symptoms of panic, replace irrational beliefs with new responses, and shut off anxious feelings instead of intensifying them.

The Major Cause of Panic

Every symptom you experience during a panic attack is a natural, harmless part of your body's fight-or-flight reaction. All panic symptoms are the direct result of the hormone adrenaline which is released by your adrenal glands when you perceive that you are in danger. Adrenaline is metabolized in your body in less than three minutes. Its effects can go away just as quickly. Therefore, if you can stop your catastrophic predictions, your panic attack will be over entirely within three minutes. This means that your anxiety need never last more than three minutes. But it is necessary to stop the loop of catastrophic thinking. The crucial step is to contest and refute any catastrophic predictions you find yourself making about your panic symptoms.

Exploring Your Fear

To prepare yourself for self-hypnosis, you will need first to look at how your panic symptoms arise. Take a moment and imagine that you are in a frightening situation. What type of situation is it? A social setting, driving a car, being around certain animals or objects, the work place, an elevator, an airplane? Now let yourself feel a little of the anxiety you would normally experience in the real situation.

Although this manufactured anxiety will differ from a full-blown panic attack, some physical symptoms may accompany it. Is your heart beating faster? Are you dizzy? Do you feel short of breath? Do your legs feel weak? Do you have difficulty swallowing? Are you hotter or colder than normal? Are you shaking or trembling? Do you have butterflies in your stomach? Do you find it hard to concentrate and think clearly? These are the most common physical symptoms of anxiety and panic. You may have some or all of them, plus other feelings unique to you.

Again imagine yourself in the same frightening situation. This time concentrate on your thoughts. Try to notice what you tell yourself about the situation and about your symptoms. Do this now.

Did you find that you make catastrophic predictions about the situation? Did you think of the worst that could possibly happen? As you began feeling anxious, did you tell yourself scary things about your symptoms of panic? Did you think that you might have a heart attack or die, that you might faint, or that you might lose control and fall down or vomit or scream? These are things that many people tell themselves during panic attacks—irrational and inaccurate predictions that prolong and intensify the panic.

Reprogramming for Results

In order to change the way your body responds to seemingly frightening situations, you need to replace your catastrophic thoughts with truthful statements that explain the nature of your symptoms: that your physical sensations won't harm you and that they will soon go away. By repeating a coping phrase that counters each symptom you notice, you will be able to realize your panic symptoms for the benign sensations that they are and start the process of lessening your fear.

You can slow your heart rate. During the fight-or-flight response, your pulse speeds up to a rate of 120 to 130 beats per minute. According to Dr. Claire Weeks, a noted authority in the field of anxiety control, the normal human heart can sustain this rate for weeks without danger. You can certainly have an elevated heart rate for a few hours without any health consequences. If you worry about your heart, get a medical checkup. Then, knowing your heart is OK, you can begin to fight your catastrophic thinking. When you feel your heart pounding, tell yourself, "My heart could beat like this for weeks and be just fine."

You can feel balanced. Feelings of dizziness or vertigo are the product of hyperventilation. It goes away when you slow down your breathing. Sometimes tension in your neck or jaw can affect your inner ear and cause dizziness. This also goes away when you relax. It is almost impossible to faint during a panic attack. The fight-or-flight reaction is actually the opposite of the fainting response. When you feel dizzy, remind yourself, "This will pass when I relax and slow my breathing."

You can breathe fully and deeply. Shortness of breath is caused by tightness in the diaphragm. This causes you to take short, quick breaths into the top of your lungs when you feel fear. The solution is to consciously take deep, slow breaths while focusing on the full exhalation of air. The coping phrase to remember is "Push the old air out. Take a new deep breath. Push the old air out. Take a new deep breath . . . " Repeat this to yourself in a slow cadence.

You can feel strength in your legs. During a panic attack your legs may feel weak. You may even fear that you will fall down. This reaction is caused by blood pooling in the veins of your thigh muscles. The fight-or-flight reaction pushes blood to your extremities to prepare you to run. The weakness you feel is an illusion, because the blood is actually making your legs ready to move, and move quickly. When blood collects in your legs in a resting state, it produces a subjective feeling of heaviness and weakness. When this happens, tell yourself, "This is just my legs preparing to run. They are stronger than usual right now."

You can swallow freely. Extensive tension in your throat may cause you to feel as though you can't swallow when you are very anxious. Actually, you could swallow if you had to. And the symptom will pass as soon as you relax. To hasten its passing, open your mouth wide and fake a yawn. Tell yourself, "I can yawn away the tension in my throat."

You can feel hot or cold and that's OK. These symptoms are caused by vasoconstriction, rising blood pressure, and changes in your sympathetic and parasympathetic nervous systems. All of these changes are a natural part of the fight-or-flight reaction and will pass when you stop making catastrophic predictions and calm down. When you feel hot or cold, tell yourself, "This will pass in a few minutes."

You can feel clear-headed. Confusion, fuzziness, and an inability to think are caused by hyperoxygenation and a high concentration of blood in your large muscles. It's all part of your body's automatic preparation for fighting or flight. These feelings can be relieved by slow, deep breathing with your mouth closed. Tell yourself, "I can just breathe deeply and slowly to clear my mind."

Repeat your coping responses to remind yourself that your symptoms are natural and harmless. You can use the self-statements recommended here or make up your own. For example, here is a complete coping statement: "My pounding heart is medically safe because my heart could beat this fast for weeks without harm. I can cope because it will pass in a few minutes." Write out each of your symptoms, why it is harmless, and how you can cope with it.

Your Total Induction

Your induction will contain a series of suggestions that will help you to:

- Relax when you are in the middle of a panic attack.
- Stop the thoughts that produced the panic attack.
- Replace the catastrophic thoughts with positive coping statements.
- Allow yourself to feel and accept all the physical sensations that accompany the attack.

RELAXATION: The induction will make use of two methods that induce physical relaxation. The first is deep breathing. With your mouth closed, take a long, slow breath into your belly. Hold it for a moment, and release it slowly and smoothly, expelling as much air as you can comfortably. Pause for a moment, pay attention to the pause, and then inhale again. The goal is slow, deep, full breaths. Deep breathing counters your body's tendency to breathe fast and shallow in the fight or flight reaction.

The second method for relaxation involves scanning your body for any areas of severe tension. Your neck and shoulders are most likely to be tense. When you find tense muscles, *will* them to relax. If you have trouble relaxing them, try making them more tense by squeezing the muscles as tightly as you can. If you can increase tension in a muscle, you can decrease tension. You may have to tense and relax your neck muscles three or four times before you get a significant reduction of residual tension.

THOUGHT-STOPPING: The induction will tell you to control catastrophic, panic-perpetuating thoughts by a technique called thought-stopping. When you start thinking that you are going to faint or that you are going to have a heart attack, you shout "STOP!" in your mind. This subvocal shout interrupts the catastrophic thought for a second. Then you quickly replace the thought with one of your coping statements, such as "It's impossible to faint—this dizziness will pass in three minutes," or "My heart is perfectly OK. It can safely pound this way for weeks, but it will slow down in three minutes."

COPING STATEMENTS: The induction will reinforce your ability to compose and use positive, factual self-statements. These are your new responses to fear. To generate an abundant supply of coping statements, begin by identifying your typical fear-producing thoughts.

You might want to keep a diary of your thoughts during stressful encounters or episodes. Whenever you feel anxious, write down your thoughts. For each irrational, fear-producing thought, write a short rebuttal. For instance, the irrational prediction "The airplane will crash" can be countered by saying: "The odds are in my favor. Airplanes almost never crash. It is safer to fly in an airplane than to drive a car." Making a realistic assessment of the odds is a good way to refute catastrophic predictions.

Another good technique for composing coping statements is to make an accurate assessment of the consequences of a feared outcome. What would happen if you did faint? What if your boss really did criticize you? What if the elevator really did get stuck for an hour? What if your date rejected your advances? Stating the likely outcome clearly will often show you that real consequences are almost never as bad as the consequences projected by your fear. It's much better to give yourself a clear view of the consequences than to leave them vague and threatening.

Distill one or two of your best coping statements into short affirmations that you can use during the induction. As you use the induction day after day, you may find that you need to alter or replace your coping statements.

ACCEPTING YOUR FEELINGS: The induction ends with two strong suggestions for accepting all your feelings and ending avoidance. The key to accepting all the feelings in your body is knowing that they are temporary. They will pass. By resisting and fighting your anxiety or panic symptoms, you get hooked into the feedback loop of ever-escalating anxiety. When you accept your feelings, no matter how painful, they pass more quickly. You soon escape the fight-or-flight discomfort.

The suggestion to end avoidance tells you that you no longer have to avoid situations, people, or things that trigger anxiety. Since you can accept, cope with, and control your feelings of fear, you can go wherever you want to go and do whatever you want to do. You will obtain a degree of freedom that up until now has remained elusive.

Using the Total Induction

Before you record your induction, make sure you have fully absorbed the concepts presented here. It's especially important to spend a sufficient amount of time examining your fear-producing thoughts and preparing your coping statements for use during the induction.

As you record your induction, follow this procedure:

1. Turn to Chapter 2 and use the *Going Down Induction*.

2. Use the *End to Anxiety Induction* at the end of this chapter. Be sure you have developed several strong coping statements that you can insert in the appropriate places.

3. Close with the *Coming Up Induction* from Chapter 2.

End to Anxiety and Panic Induction

Let yourself drift deeper and deeper . . . deeper and deeper, drifting and drowsy, drowsy and drifting. Drifting down, down, down, into total relaxation. Drifting deeper and deeper, deeper and deeper. You feel safe and relaxed. You are aware now that symptoms of anxiety are your body's natural fight-or-flight response. They are natural and harmless. They are unimportant, they are unimportant. And you are losing your fear of the symptoms of anxiety. You are unafraid of the symptoms of anxiety. They are your body's natural fight-or-flight response. You accept the harmless symptoms of anxiety. You remind yourself that you are medically safe. Right now you remind yourself of what your symptoms mean and why you are medically safe. [PAUSE 15 SECONDS.] *Whatever your symptoms, you know they are unimportant and that you are medically safe. Your symptoms are natural, you are losing your fear of the symptoms of anxiety. You are becoming stronger, more confident, more self-assured. You are in control of your fears and anxieties.*

You can relax your body whenever you feel fear or panic, you can breathe deeply, deeply. The air will push deep into your abdomen . . . deep down into your belly. Take a deep breath into your belly . . . and let go. Exhale that old air. You can take slow, deep breaths to regulate your breathing . . . deep breaths into your belly, slowly letting go. Whenever you feel anxious you can begin taking slow, deep breaths into your abdomen. Take another deep breath to remind yourself that you can regulate your breathing . . . you will breathe slowly, deeply, whenever you feel anxious. You can relax your whole body. When you are anxious you can check your body for tension. You will check your shoulders and neck, letting your shoulders droop and relax. You will check your jaw, letting your jaw hang loosely, loosely. You will check your forehead, letting it become smooth, smooth and relaxed. You will check your abdomen, letting each deep breath relax your stomach, each deep breath relaxing your stomach more and more deeply. You can relax any part of your body that feels tension. When you are anxious, you will check and relax any tension area in your body. You know that you are in charge. You have the tools and knowledge to let go of all anxiety and fear.

You know the truth now, that panic passes quickly when you stop your anxious thoughts. Panic passes quickly. It passes in less than three minutes when you empty your mind of anxious thoughts. You can wait it out and soon, very soon, it will be over. When you are feeling anxiety and panic you can stop the anxious thoughts, stop the thoughts of danger. Inside your mind you will shout "STOP!" to the anxious thoughts, knowing your panic will pass in less than three minutes. You can shout "STOP!" inside your mind to cease the anxious thoughts. Panic passes quickly, it is over, over, over. Panic passes and it's over when you stop the anxious thoughts. You can wait it out and soon the panic will be over. You are in charge, you have the ability to release all panic and anxious thoughts.

Imagine your anxiety as a picture hanging in a museum, perhaps a picture of war or strife or anguish. See the picture on the wall of the museum. You are moving past the picture, floating past the picture, you are almost past the picture . . . and now it disappears from sight. Your anxiety passes like the picture out of sight, out of sight. You know now that you can accept any feeling in your body. You can accept any emotion because you float past, float past, float past, until it is gone and out of sight. You accept and float past your feelings.

Now you have new responses to your old anxious thoughts. You no longer frighten yourself with the catastrophic fears. You are letting go of the old fear, the old anxiety . . . letting go, letting go, letting go of the old fears. Right now you can remind yourself of your new responses to the old anxious thoughts. [PAUSE 15 SECONDS.] Whenever you are aware of the old anxious thoughts, you know now that you can stop them. Those thoughts are fading, fading, fading. See them fading like a light going out in the distance. You have new responses to the old anxious thoughts.

You know now that you can accept any feeling in your body. You can accept any emotion. You accept without running from your feelings and emotions. You accept without running. You float past anxiety and panic, knowing it is a brief time and in a while you will feel so much better. You float past without fighting. You know now your feelings are transient and passing . . . they are passing, passing and soon will be gone. Your feelings, no matter how uncomfortable, pass and are gone. They are gone. Your anxiety or panic soon will be gone. You accept and float past your feelings.

You are becoming stronger, stronger . . . more and more confident. You are stronger and more confident because you accept and let feelings pass. You embrace your feelings, both painful and pleasurable, because they pass and are soon gone. You have nothing to fear because they pass and are soon gone. You have nothing to fear because you accept your feelings. You are hopeful and confident. You are able now to cope with your feelings, you can relax and cope. See yourself walking tall and straight, see the strength in your step. You accept the future without worry because you can cope with panic and anxiety. You can cope and float past panic. In three minutes the panic will be over if you relax and take slow deep breaths, if you empty your mind of anxious thoughts. In three minutes, any panic will be over if you float past, letting go of anxious thoughts.

And now you will be able to enter any situations where you once felt stressed. You can enter because you accept your feelings, you can cope with your feelings. You go wherever you want and you do whatever you want because you are confident in your ability to cope. You know now that you can enter any situation and remember your coping skills. You have new abilities to cope and you feel a growing confidence in your abilities to cope. You can enter any situation because you can float past your fear . . . letting go, letting go, letting go . . . feeling so strong, so confident. You are in charge, you are able to cope with any stressful situations. You feel very relaxed, very peaceful. And in a few moments you will come back to full conscious awareness, feeling stronger and more positive . . . feeling confident and strong. And in a few moments you will come back up from one to ten. You will come all the way up feeling alert, refreshed, and wide awake. You will feel completely alert and awake. You will feel relaxed and renewed when you come all the way up. And you are starting to come up.

The Companion Induction
to End Panic and Anxiety

You have now learned to accept, cope with, and control your feelings of fear and anxiety by using the *Hypnosis to End Panic and Anxiety Induction.* You may want to add a booster shot to your recovery by including the following *Companion Induction* which will help strengthen your goals. The imagery in the induction will create a new blueprint for your subconscious mind—one that will reinforce positive behavior and feelings long after you have recovered from your fears and anxieties.

How to use the Companion Induction

1. Turn to Chapter 2. Use the *Going Down Induction.*

2. Insert the *Companion Induction.*

3. Turn to Chapter 2. Use the *Coming Up Induction*.

4. The *Companion Induction* can be used in conjunction with the *Hypnosis to End Anxiety and Panic Induction*.

The Companion Induction to End Anxiety and Panic

Now just imagine that some time has passed, a day or two, perhaps a week or a month. See yourself in the near future. Imagine that you have made tremendous progress. You have let go of the old fears, old anxieties. You now have new coping skills, new tools that give you control over your anxieties and stresses. Each day you grow stronger, more confident, more self-assured. You can cope with any situation regardless of how stressful. You have practiced your new techniques and have stopped panic attacks before they had a chance to start. Many of the old fears are far behind you and are fading more and more each day. This image of the future is your new blueprint. Bring it to the present moment and it will begin to manifest itself and grow stronger and stronger each day. Now, imagine for a moment that you have just stopped a panic attack by using your new skills. You breathe easy, you feel steady, your chest and stomach are calm. You have succeeded, you have accomplished your goal. You have won. You have control. The feeling is wonderful. You feel proud of yourself, you feel a great sense of confidence. You know that you can do it. Imagine a smile on your face. See yourself standing tall. You enjoy life now without all the old fears. They are just old baggage from the past. You have let them go. You are able to cope with any situations regardless of how stressful they may be. You float through them. You just float through them. Let them go. Let them fade, fade, fade away. You have strength, confidence, you are in charge of your life. Now conclude your imagery by seeing yourself in your special place and reflect on all of your new and powerful feelings of confidence, trusting yourself to cope with any situation, and liking who you are. Just enjoy these positive feelings for a few more minutes.

17

Healing the Adult
Survivor of Child Abuse

"My father beat me when he got drunk, and he got drunk a lot. But what does that have to do with my inability to stay in a relationship or make commitments?"

"My father and uncle both sexually abused me from the age of five years old. I lived in terror of these two men for most of my childhood. Even though I've been married three times, I still find it impossible to trust my mate and difficult to tolerate sexual intercourse."

"I lack confidence and don't feel very good about myself. As a child I don't remember my parents ever approving of anything I did."

These are common statements from people who have been abused in some way as children. Child abuse is often accepted as normal behavior within the family, especially if at least one parent was abused as a child. The severity of abuse can vary widely. Bed without supper can be as painful and frightening as being locked inside a closet. Even a loud, stinging "should" can hurt as though it were a slap across the face. When does well-meaning discipline become abuse? The question is difficult to answer, but the result of childhood punishment can last a lifetime.

The Abusive Home

Three environmental factors are often associated with child abuse.

The Alcoholic Family. Heavy drinking or drug abuse is often a prevalent part of the home life that surrounds child abuse. According to specialists in the field, alcohol, drugs, or both are usually present when physical or sexual abuse occurs. These substances cause boundaries and limits to blur or disappear. In many cases family members hide their dependency. Children in alcoholic families are left to guess the cause of their parents' strange behavior. Often these children blame themselves. The following descriptions of substance-addicted behavior may help you determine whether alcohol or drugs influenced the actions of adults in your family.

• Drastic changes in personality
• Erratic mood swings
• Displays of anger or overzealous affection
• Loss of memory
• Chronic depression
• Use of alcohol or drugs to relieve stress
• Loss of physical coordination

Emotional Dysfunction. When a parent is disconnected from his or her feelings or when certain feelings are denied or disallowed in a family, it is virtually impossible to create an environment that encourages trust, nurturing, and the freedom to grow and create. Children soon learn to hide their feelings and to expect very little parental support. The family may seem perfectly balanced to the outside world, but hidden and unexpressed emotions erode trust and normal bonding within the family unit.

Abusive Family History. In one family the father lined up his children once a year for their annual spanking—whether they needed it or not. He used a switch. Once grown, his daughter used a hairbrush on her children; his daughter's son used a wooden paddle on his. The pattern is repeated from one generation to the next. Whatever the form of abuse, it will reoccur until the cycle is finally healed and stopped.

Owning the Pain

There are three categories of abuse: physical, sexual, and emotional. In many cases physical or sexual abuse is obvious and the trauma it causes apparent. However, the grown victim often masks the memory of suffering by adopting defense mechanisms such as denial and amnesia. Often, especially when emotional abuse is involved, the damage can be covert and therefore go unrecognized as abuse. You may not think of yourself as having been an abused child, but wonder why you now suffer from low self-esteem or lack of confidence or why you feel fearful, have an eating disorder, or choose abusive, unnurturing partners.

The first step in healing the wounds of child abuse is to recognize the fact that you did suffer abuse as a child. Often the memory is so completely buried that your only clue to the trauma will be certain behavioral similarities that you share with other survivors of abuse. The following sections describe the different types of abuse and the possible behavior patterns they can elicit.

Physical Abuse. Georgette had several different stepfathers throughout her childhood, and all of them thought that a good beating was the best way to discipline a child. Whenever Georgette behaved in a way that made her noticeable to any of her stepfathers, she received a sound beating with a brush, belt, or switch. Since slightly different versions of the same type of behavior were required to arouse the anger of each stepfather, Georgette never knew when certain actions would draw someone's wrath. With very little control over her life, Georgette rebelled by finding something she could take charge of—her body weight. Georgette soon became obsessed with keeping her weight dangerously low and eventually began to use laxatives to rid her body of what she had eaten. She discovered that vomiting after meals would increase weight loss. This destructive act became addictive, and soon Georgette could not stop from purging her food.

Today Georgette is 45 and looks well over 50. She begins each meal with something colorful like a tomato. This distinctive tracer comes up last when Georgette purges her food and tells her when to stop vomiting. Georgette is a creative, intelligent woman, yet she has very little confidence and her self-image is completely distorted. She has attempted suicide twice. Unable to work, Georgette sees herself as a complete failure. She is now in a support group that helps her deal with her early abuse so that she can regain her self-worth and physical well-being.

Any form of physical abuse leaves emotional scars that far outlast the wound itself. Since physical abuse can have long-term devastating effects, most child psychologists believe that no physical punishment should ever be inflicted.

In many cases of severe physical abuse children will find ways to protect themselves. One method of defensive action is mental escape into fantasy. Abused children may pretend that the torture is not taking place. They may remove themselves from the scene mentally and cling to an imaginary world where pain doesn't exist. Or, in order to find the refuge they so desperately need, physically abused children may withdraw deeply within themselves to a place where no one can reach them. This is one type of defense. Here is a list of other behavioral and emotional characteristics that may arise from childhood physical abuse.

- Trouble identifying reality (unrealistically high or low expectations of people, assuming people don't like you)
- Fear of letting people get to know the "real you" (you think they'll discover some awful hidden flaw)
- Inability to feel or express love and affection
- Belief that a subpersonality or monster within you will leap out and be destructive
- Feeling ashamed (blaming yourself for the abusive behavior of your parents)
- Masking your real feelings
- Feeling sudden bursts of anger and aggressive impulses
- Feeling unworthy and avoiding challenges

Sexual Abuse. At 35, Karen is a successful accountant for a large public relations firm. She is happily married and has two daughters aged three and five. Karen has spent many years in therapy recovering from sexual abuse by her mother and brother.

Karen's father spent very little time with his family and therefore was unaware that any problems existed. Her mother drank heavily and sexually abused and beat her children when she was drunk. She seduced her oldest son first and then coerced her son to join her as she sexually abused the two younger girls. The abuse lasted for many years. Karen and her sister viewed their brother as an obese monster and their mother as a cruel witch. The young sisters helped each other to survive by pretending that they were being held captive in a huge castle. They survived their ordeal but were left with deep psychological wounds.

Karen has regained her self-esteem and improved her sexual relationship with her husband. However, Karen is still plagued with a tremendous fear that she may turn into her mother and beat and abuse her own daughters. Her fear is so strong that she denies her daughters any physical contact. She feels afraid to hug them, kiss them, and hold them.

Sexual abuse is not always easy to identify. When parents flirt or tell sexual stories or touch their children in inappropriate ways, these abusive behaviors can be disguised as love and affection. The more indistinguishable sexual abuse is, the more confusing it is to a child. A child experiences conflicts between feeling invaded and loved. When limitations are relaxed and boundaries are crossed, a child is robbed of the natural progression of sexual development.

As an adult, the survivor of sexual abuse may find it hard to have normal relationships. Some of the problems can be:

- Intense sex drive
- Low sex drive
- Inability to have lasting sexual relationships
- Fear of intimacy
- Fear of sex
- Fear of men or women
- Feelings of intimidation with present or potential sexual partners
- Choosing abusive partners
- Choosing withdrawing partners

Emotional Abuse. At 29, Robert sets foot outside his apartment once every two days. He forces himself through the door, down the street, and into the grocery store. If he sees someone walking toward him, he'll cross the street and continue walking on the other side. He isn't afraid that the stranger will hurt him; he's afraid that he will say hello and that Robert will then have to respond. The thought of such an encounter can make Robert's heart beat fast as his breath becomes shallow. If Robert could recognize his thoughts at this point, he would be able to give voice to his fear: "This person won't like me. They won't think that I'm enough. I'll disappoint them." From an objective viewpoint, this fear seems irrational. It makes little sense that a stranger's potential acceptance or rejection can affect Robert's behavior so severely. But to Robert his fear is very real, and it runs his life every day.

Although he couldn't voice it at the time, as a child Robert never felt accepted or actually loved by either of his parents. His father, a chemist, spent most of his time either at the lab or in his study at home. He was constantly occupied with work and left the matter of Robert's upbringing to his wife. Robert's mother had a very strong sense of what was right and wrong and she tried to instill this moral code in Robert at a very young age. According to his mother's ethics, feelings showed weakness, and so they topped the long list of taboo topics of conversation. Robert quickly got the message; if you had a feeling, you were deeply deficient in some very important way. Robert did have feelings, but he never admitted this to anyone.

Robert's mother had feelings too. Had she been able to recognize and admit them, she would have known that she felt very bitter. And that the bitterness was directed towards the man she had married— who by now had completely withdrawn from her. Robert could sense his mother's bitterness, but since he couldn't ask about it or seek reassurance, he thought her anger was directed at him. As a result, Robert developed the belief that he would always disappoint others.

Emotional abuse may seem less traumatic or less noticeable, but it can do enormous harm. This type of abuse often goes undetected because much of it is nonverbal. Certain facial expressions or nuances in voice tone can make a lasting impression. Think of the familiar expression "All my mother had to do was look at me in a certain way and I knew I'd better shape up." In healthy families, discipline is balanced with love, compassion, and kindness. Without this healthy balance, a stern look can feel like a beating, a sharp word like abandonment.

There are certain abusive dynamics that occur in families that are emotionally dysfunctional. Here are some examples.

- Neglect. Your parents were too preoccupied with themselves to notice you. Or your parents disapproved of something you did or didn't do and withheld love as punishment.
- Inconsistency. The family was chaotic and the rules changed daily. What was acceptable one day might not hold true the next.
- Disapproval. No matter what you did or how hard you tried, it wasn't good enough. If you received an A in math, and a B in geography, you should have received an A in both. When you did do well, your parents took credit for it. "Of course you won the tennis match. You're my child, aren't you?" your parent might say. "When I played I won more matches than anyone else on the team."
- Guilt. Your parents may have manipulated and controlled you by inflicting guilt. You felt shamed into doing what you may not have wanted to do or felt right doing. Feeling guilty is an emotion that can rob you of your self-esteem and confidence.
- Fear and intimidation. Your parents may have created an emotional environment that threatened your safety. Impending violence, disaster, or punishment takes away all sense of security. This potential threatening outcome can be broadcast through body language and gestures.

Self-Discovery Chart

As an adult, you may experience feelings and emotions that you cannot explain. They may nag at you or depress you. They may be chronic or occur sporadically. The following self-discovery chart may help you to determine if abuse was present in your childhood. The conditions listed are common among survivors of abuse. Check the ones that apply to you.

[ ] Fear of letting people get to know the "real you" (you think they'll discover some awful hidden flaw)

[ ] Fear of being controlled, engulfed or emotionally suffocated by others

[ ] Fear that you will become uncontrollably destructive

[ ] Fear of rejection and abandonment

[ ] Fear of intimacy

[ ] Fear of expressing your needs

[ ] Feeling ashamed (blaming yourself for the abusive behavior of your parents)

[ ] Feeling sudden bursts of anger and aggressive impulses

[ ] Feeling unworthy and avoiding challenges

[ ] Feeling guilty for not meeting your own expectations or those of others

[ ] Feeling intimidated by or hostile toward authority figures

[ ] Feeling intimidated by present or potential sexual partners

[ ] Masking your real feelings

[ ] Inability to feel or express love and affection

[ ] Inability to maintain lasting relationships

[ ] Choosing abusive or abnormally withdrawn partners

[ ] Intense or low sex drive

[ ] Perfectionism (compulsion to always do the right thing)

[ ] Addictions (excessive use of cigarettes, alcohol, drugs or food)

[ ] Trouble identifying reality (unrealistic expectations of people, assuming people don't like you)

[ ] Control (a need to control the behavior, feelings, and responses of significant people in your life)

If you checked several of these conditions, you may want to explore the possibility that you were abused as a child. In order to develop a greater sense of self-worth, learn to trust in others, and gain peace of heart and mind, a survivor of child abuse needs to undergo a twofold process. First, old patterns of thought that now hinder your quest for growth need to be replaced by new, positive affirmations. This will allow you to learn new ways to live your life. Second, the child who was wounded by abuse needs to be contacted and held and taken care of by you, the adult of the present. This healing will make it possible for you to let go of the pain that persists in the present and inhibits your ability to love and trust.

Reprogramming Old Patterns

The Self-Discovery Chart illustrates some issues that are common to survivors of child abuse. The conditions you checked have probably been with you for such a long time that they have become habits. Habits are feelings or thoughts that have been programmed into your subconscious mind and result in reoccurring behavior. In order to change negative behavioral patterns, you must change the ways you view yourself. For example, if you think of yourself as shy and unable to go out on a date, you probably won't date. If you think of yourself as a klutz, you will probably continue to trip over your dog. But if you begin to give yourself positive messages like "I am a wonderful, loving, fun person," or "I am graceful, coordinated and agile," you will increase your chances for a date and your dog will love you. Please note that it is not necessary for your intellect to believe your new messages, because the subconscious is the part of your mind that you are trying to persuade. If you persistently repeat affirmative messages, the subconscious will often let go of some of your old programming, thereby allowing new feelings and behaviors to take root.

New Messages: Take a look at the issues you checked on the Self-Discovery Chart. Write them down here, listing them in order of priority.

1. _____

2. _____

3. _____

4. _____

5. _____

Now you are ready to create your new messages. Look at the first issue that you've written down. Think of a specific instance in your life in which this type of feeling or behavior significantly hampers you. For example, let's say the most debilitating issue for you is fear of intimacy. Try to think of a way in which you behave that directly results from your fear of intimacy. If this is really a difficult issue for you, your mind may not want to fix steadily on the problem, and as you try to become more specific, you may come up with blanks. That's OK. Persistently return your focus to the original question until you think of one way that your fear of intimacy affects your daily behavior. You might say, "Because I fear intimacy, I never initiate a conversation with a stranger." Now probe a little deeper. Try to get in touch with the *specific* fear that underlies the behavior. You may say, "I never start a conversation with a stranger because I'm afraid I'll make a fool of myself." You now have a specific problem you can work with. Remember, this statement doesn't have to penetrate the core of the issue. You needn't solve the whole problem all at once. Chipping away at the problem bit by bit is more than sufficient.

Next, define the way in which you would like to be seen by a stranger in conversation. Fascinating? Intelligent? Caring? Perceptive?

Once you've identified how you would like to be seen, you can write your new positive message. It may go like this: "I am an intelligent, perceptive human being and I feel confident in my ability to convey my ideas to others." Here are more possible ways to work with some of the other main issues.

1. If the issue is perfectionism, define the problem specifically. It may be "When I make a mistake, I'm afraid that others will laugh at me." The new message could then read, "Mistakes are for learning and growing. I am a good person who can make mistakes. It's natural and human to make mistakes. I accept both my mistakes and my achievements."
2. If the issue is that you are intimidated by authority figures, a specific problem could be "I get so nervous when I'm around persons in authority that I don't know what to say to them." The new message might then be "I am a worthwhile person. I feel confident and self-assured around authority figures."
3. If the issue is that you feel guilty for not meeting someone else's expectations, the specific problem could be "I feel so guilty when my husband complains about something around the house." The new message could read, "I have done the best I can and I feel good about myself. I've done well with many responsibilities."

Make sure the new messages are stated as positives. Never put the word *not* in an hypnotic suggestion. The statement "I *won't* let others make me feel bad" can be confusing to your subconscious and should be rephrased as "I feel confident and good about myself with others."

Now make a list of the old patterns and write the new messages beside them.

OLD PATTERNS   NEW MESSAGES

1. _____   _____
   _____   _____
2. _____   _____
   _____   _____
3. _____   _____
   _____   _____
4. _____   _____
   _____   _____
5. _____   _____
   _____   _____

Programming for Results

Now that you have clearly stated all of your new messages, you are ready to incorporate them into your subconscious. The *New Messages Induction* that follows will help you become more confident and increase your self esteem. Your new messages will become your new patterns of thought, feeling, and behavior.

Build confidence to release negative patterns. The induction suggests that you "Let yourself imagine being more confident. Each day you come closer and closer to your goals, each day you release and let go of old patterns, old negative patterns that have only held you back."

Recall a positive experience to increase self worth. The induction suggests that you recall and "Imagine a time that you felt good about an accomplishment, or a goal you obtained, or a compliment that you received. Remember that good feeling, recall that good feeling . . . recall all the wonderful details around that special event." Even the smallest success can conjure up good feelings about yourself, thereby improving your sense of self worth.

Inserting your new messages. At this juncture the induction gives you the opportunity to insert your new messages, such as "When someone compliments me, I say thank you and feel that I deserve it" or "I am a worthwhile person. I feel confident and self-assured with everyone I meet." To maximize the power of your messages, limit them to five per induction. You can use the same messages repeatedly or replace them with new ones. You can judge your progress by how quickly your new messages take effect.

Anchoring the new messages. In order to give your new messages strength, the induction suggests: "Imagine your new messages taking root. You look and feel more confident, more self-assured. You like yourself, you are proud of yourself, you are admired and respected by your friends and family. Your new messages are taking hold, growing stronger and stronger." The more positive emotions you can elicit from these hypnotic suggestions, the more your new messages will be anchored into your subconscious.

Using the Induction

The *New Messages Induction* should be inserted between the two parts of *The Relaxation Induction* in Chapter 2. You may want to tape the total induction keeping in mind the following procedure:

1. Turn to Chapter 2. Use the *Going Down Induction*.

2. Use The *New Messages Induction* which follows. Remember to write your new

messages in the space provided prior to using the induction.

3. Turn to Chapter 2. Use the *Coming Up Induction.*

4. Use the induction daily until the old patterns are replaced with your new messages.

The New Messages Induction

Now just enjoy your special place, let yourself drift and float, deeper and deeper, feeling so comfortable, so relaxed. Let a feeling of total peace move through your entire body. You feel as though all of your goals and desires are becoming more and more attainable. Let yourself imagine being more confident, more confident. Each moment, each day you come closer and closer to your goals. Each moment, each day you release and let go of old patterns, old negative patterns that have only held you back, old negative patterns that have only caused you stress. You let them go, release them and let them go. Just see them in your mind's eye, and see them just fade [PAUSE], just fade [PAUSE]. Let them go, let feelings of peace flow through your body. Let feelings of confidence grow stronger and stronger as you watch old negative patterns fade, fade, fade. A stronger feeling of confidence grows, you feel better and better about yourself. Now just imagine a time that you felt good about an accomplishment, or a goal you obtained, or a compliment you received. Remember that good feeling, recall that good feeling, experience that feeling of accomplishment. [PAUSE.] Imagine that smile on your face, or that feeling of pride. Just recall all the wonderful details around that special event. [PAUSE.] Now keep these feelings, hold on to them, let these feelings of confidence grow, feeling better and better about yourself. Now just continue to relax and at this point insert your new messages [SUCH AS: *"When someone compliments me, I say thank you and feel that I deserve it. "* OR *"I am a worthwhile person. I feel confident and self-assured with everyone I meet"*]. *Write your own new messages here:*

_____

_____

_____

_____

Now just imagine your new messages taking root. You look and feel more confident, more self-assured. You like yourself, you are proud of yourself, you are a wonderful person, you deserve the very best. You are admired and respected by your friends and family, you are becoming more and more confident, your new messages are taking hold, growing stronger and stronger. Now let all of these positive feelings and images go deep into your subconscious, growing stronger and stronger. Just drift for another moment, and let your mind slowly return to your special place, your special place of peace and calm.

The Abused Child Within

Have you ever been near someone and noticed that something about them—their smile, their gait, their fragrance—reminds you of your second-grade teacher? At that moment, a whole sequence of memories may come flooding back—the classroom with its hardwood floors, the sound of the recess bell, the kids yelling in the school yard. Many things can trigger memories from your childhood. When you are in touch with these memories and the feelings they evoke, you are in touch with your inner child.

For the survivor of child abuse, these feelings are often less benign than those in the example. Hurt, anger, fear, and shame may all enter a painful, vivid memory. But in spite of the pain that exists, a part of your inner child still loves to play and is very clear about what you want and what you need in your life. When thoughts emerge like "I don't want to do that," or "I'm not listening," you are hearing the voice of your inner child.

The effect that the inner child can have on adult behavior is documented in studies by Jung, Freud, and numerous others. More recently Charles L. Whitfield, M.D., wrote *Healing the Child Within*, W. Hugh Missildine offered *Your Inner Child of the Past*, and Buck S. Fonvard wrote *Betrayal of Innocence*. Many studies agree that in order to heal past wounds you need to connect with and heal your inner child.

Meeting Your Inner Child

Close your eyes for a moment, take a breath of air, and relax. Now let an image of a child emerge. It may be a vulnerable infant, a playful child of eight, or a rebellious teenager. If it is too difficult to create an image, try recalling a familiar photograph. At times you may see an image that does not look as you looked when you were a child. That's fine. The image you conjure will act as a symbol of your inner child. It doesn't have to look exactly like you.

Healing Your Inner Child

The *Inner Child Induction* will suggest that you imagine a special place at which you will meet your inner child. Visualize a safe and peaceful place for your meeting. Your inner child needs to feel safe and secure. In this special place, you can ask your inner child questions such as "What can I do to help you feel better? What do you need? What information can you give me?" After you ask each question, stop, wait, and listen. The answers may not come immediately. In fact, the induction may have to be repeated several times before your inner child feels safe enough to say anything. In addition to listening to what your inner child has to say, notice the expression on his or her face, and what emotions your inner child is displaying. Be aware of his or her body language. Is your inner child withdrawn or open? It is perfectly fine for you and your inner child not to talk to each other. Learning to be comfortable in the other's presence need not require words.

When you have concluded your conversation with your inner child, take a moment to reflect on the love that exists in your life—the love you have for your own child, mate, friends, or favorite pet. Direct that love to your inner child, embrace him or her, and let your inner child know that he or she is important. The induction suggests that you let these wonderful feelings bond you and your inner child together so that healing can begin to take place.

Using the Inner Child Induction

Now that you have an understanding of the components that are built into your induction, you are ready to record it. Follow these steps:

1. Turn to Chapter 2 and use the *Going Down Induction*.

2. Use the *Healing the Inner Child Induction*.

3. Turn to Chapter 2 and record the *Coming Up Induction*.

Healing the Inner Child Induction

Now just imagine allowing your inner child to enter your special place, which is so peaceful, so loving, so safe, so secure, and now just imagine your inner child appearing to you. [PAUSE 30 SECONDS.] *Now notice what your inner child looks like. What is your inner child wearing? What expression is on your inner child's face? Is your inner child happy or sad? Now notice your inner child's body language. Is your inner child open or closed? Make friends with your inner child. Let your inner child know he or she is safe, wanted, and important.* [PAUSE 30 SECONDS.] *Now you can ask your inner child some questions if you like, such as, "What can I do to help you feel better? What are your needs? What information do you need to give me?" Now ask your questions and wait patiently for the answers. Be sure you listen to your inner child. It may take a while for the answers to come and that's fine. If your inner child chooses not to talk with you, that's fine, too. Just be together enjoying your safe and special place.* [PAUSE AS MUCH TIME AS YOU NEED.] *Begin to conclude your visit and as you do so reflect for a moment on the love that you possess—the love you have for your own child, mate, friends, or favorite pet.* [PAUSE 20 SECONDS.] *Let yourself feel that love and warmth and affection. And now direct that love, warmth, and affection toward your inner child. Embrace your inner child, hold your child, let your child know how important he or she is. Acknowledge your inner child's existence, and as you communicate your feelings of love, warmth, and nurturing, let the feelings join you together and feel a healing taking place. A healing that flows through you completely. And now just enjoy your special place as a wonderful healing takes place. Let yourself feel reconnected with your inner child, whole, in harmony with your mind, body, and spirit.* [PAUSE AS LONG AS YOU NEED.] *Before you return, let your inner child know that you will be seeing him or her again and ask whether your child has any last messages for you.* [PAUSE . . . AS LONG AS YOU NEED.] *Now just continue to relax and enjoy your special place.*

What to Expect and Following Up

Use the *Healing the Inner Child Induction* daily for about a month. When you feel a significant change taking place, you may want to reduce your use of the induction to one or two times a week. It is important that you continue improving your self-esteem and confidence at the same time. You may want to alternate the *Inner Child Induction* with the *Self-Esteem Induction* in Chapter 11.

Recovery is a process that will dip and curve, regress and progress. One day you may feel great and think you have gotten rid of the old problems, and the next day they may return. With continual use of the induction, you will notice that the rough edges are softening and the low times are easier to handle.

Case Study

Helena was an attractive, tall, platinum blonde woman who at age 55 had achieved great success as president of her own marketing firm. She was beautiful, intelligent, and stylish. Outwardly, her life seemed full and rewarding. Within, things were different. Although she had reached many goals, feelings of failure, depression, and worthlessness plagued her. Her depression drove her to several suicide attempts.

She had spent many years in psychotherapy and knew the origin of her feelings. As early as she could remember, she felt as if her mother did not want her. Her mother continuously reinforced her daughter's feelings by telling her that she never wanted Helena to be born, that she was too much of a financial burden.

At age twelve, Helena withdrew emotionally. She no longer felt any pain, and she no longer felt love. Consequently, as an adult she had great difficulty expressing her feelings, or even knowing what they were. She could not relate intimately and had very few friends.

Helena sought hypnotherapy as a means to reach her emotions and rid herself of depression and negative behavior. She had one session per week for two months. In her third session, during the *Healing the Inner Child Induction,* she visualized meeting the twelve-year-old who had shut her feelings down. She talked with her, asking how she could help her heal. The child responded that she wanted to be acknowledged as a worthwhile person. She wanted to go to the park and play. Helena visualized taking her to the park, having a picnic, and enjoying each other's company.

In essence, Helena became the child's mother and treated her as she would like to have been treated by her own mother. As Helena visualized nurturing and loving her inner child, she felt a healing taking place. In another session Helena met herself as an infant. She saw herself lying in the crib, alone, lonely, and rejected. Helena picked up and embraced the infant, and while she held the child she began to cry. As she wept she released some of the sadness of her past. At the end of the two-month program, she had released her depression and suicidal thoughts. She was happier, felt more confident, and was able to better understand her mother's issues and emotional problems.

Special Considerations

Once you begin to explore the areas of your childhood abuse, you may feel like you are opening Pandora's Box. You may not be prepared to see what is in there. The most productive plan is to find a qualified therapist who is familiar with childhood abuse and can act as a guide and adviser.

18

Loss and Separation

Nancy looks at the pile of boxes she has yet to unpack, but a feeling of isolation paralyzes her good intentions. She feels lonely and far away from home.

Kurt hangs up the phone frustrated and angry with his ex-wife. They can't seem to resolve their differences. He misses his children and feels stuck. The same problems keep repeating themselves with no solution in sight.

Richard's company reorganized and terminated his department, leaving him without a job after many years of good service. He feels rejected and betrayed. His life has been disrupted and his financial security threatened.

Although Nancy, Kurt, and Richard each have experienced a different type of loss, they share similar emotions. Whenever you have to let go of something you love, depend on, or are just accustomed to, you experience a separation reaction. The following are some statements that describe the emotional impact of loss:

"I feel anxious and worried when he doesn't call. I can't concentrate on anything."

"I feel angry. Why did she leave me? I don't know if I can manage by myself."

"I feel stuck. I just keep thinking about the problem over and over and over."

"I'm lonely and sad. My friends are far away."

"I feel depressed. The dream is lost and I can't seem to get over it."

It is important to remember that these emotions are part of the separation reaction and, in fact, will help you heal. Denying or suppressing your feelings will only delay recovery.

Types of Loss

Emotions associated with the separation reaction occur whenever your lifestyle changes significantly. Some of the situations which can cause a separation reaction are:

Divorce or separation from your family. The trauma of a split in a long-term marriage can be devastating to an entire family. Even the couple's friends will be affected by the separation.

Job loss. Losing financial security and the camaraderie of co-workers often result in feelings of low self-esteem and loss of confidence.

Loss of a dream. The loss of nearly anything you have anticipated or hoped for triggers a separation reaction. When a child is disabled or disadvantaged in some way, hopes that the parents have built up for many years may suddenly be destroyed or compromised. Feelings of helplessness and frustration can invade all areas of the family's life.

Moving to a new location. Although the move may be to a better job or a larger home, the loss of good friends, old neighbors, and perhaps a well-loved home may cause feelings of loneliness and abandonment to arise.

Completion of a project. Finishing a manuscript or reaching a long-term goal, such as obtaining a degree, can be anticlimactic. Feelings of loss, depression, or confusion may suddenly well up.

Loss of mobility or health. Health and well-being may suddenly be lost due to injury or illness. This type of loss makes participation in sports and other enjoyable activities impossible.

Loss of a precious object. Although the value of the loss may be covered by insurance, nothing can ever replace the true worth of a great grandmother's wedding ring or the coins collected since childhood.

Rejection. When relations are severed with a good friend or lover, sadness, anger, and hurt can become predominant emotions.

Physical Symptoms of the Separation Reaction

When your thoughts and emotions are joyful and light, your body feels strong, vibrant, and healthy. Recall now an extremely happy moment. Perhaps you kissed your sweetheart good night and went home whistling, skipping, and dancing down the street. You felt as though you were floating a foot off the ground. The same holds true when thoughts become depressed, fearful, or angry. Your entire body reacts. Possible physical symptoms include:

- **Insomnia.** You may have a hard time falling asleep or you may wake suddenly in the middle of the night and can't get back to sleep.
- **Fatigue.** You may sleep longer hours during the night but awaken feeling exhausted.
- **Change in eating patterns.** You may lose your appetite or overeat.
- **Throat, chest, and stomach constriction.** You may find it hard to swallow. Your chest may feel tight and your stomach may feel as if a swarm of butterflies inside it are beating their wings in unison.
- **Anxiety attacks.** You may experience shortness of breath, clammy hands, or heart palpitations.

You might experience one or more of the symptoms described. These physical reactions to loss can certainly feel bad and sometimes threatening, but most of the time they are harmless. You should, however, always consult your physician to rule out a medical condition as the cause.

The Five Stages of Recovery

All things continuously change and transform. Just when you become comfortable with one set of circumstances, life can throw you a curve and important people or things in your life may be lost. Again you must readjust. The emotional adjustments in a separation reaction can be divided into five stages. As each stage is completed, you transcend to a stronger state of well-being. Although many people experience the stages of recovery in the sequence listed, these stages may be experienced in almost any order. It's also not uncommon for one stage to reoccur in a cyclical manner. The two stages most likely to be repeated are the realization stage and the immobilization stage. When this happens it's an indication that you are holding on to emotions generated by your loss instead of letting the recovery process unfold. Here are the five stages.

COPING. Your loss may come as suddenly and unexpectedly as the loss of a job or abandonment by your spouse. If this happens, all of your energy will be directed toward self-preservation. Issues such as "Can I provide for the kids?" and "Will the money be there?" become central to your thoughts and actions. You find ways to cope with the immediate needs that your loss demands.

REALIZATION. Once you have regained some equilibrium, there is an awakening that occurs. Now you begin to realize the full impact of your loss. Life is in an upheaval and it may never be the same again. In this stage, you may experience mood swings that include anger, depression, and fear.

IMMOBILIZATION. This is a stage of emotional paralysis. You may feel stuck, unable to let it go, and find it difficult to move beyond your loss. You may replay the separation over and over in your mind. You may feel victimized and powerless. You may feel responsible and wish to go back and undo the event that caused the loss.

ACCEPTANCE. This is not a state of total recovery. It is another phase. It is a time when the emotional pain is reduced. In the acceptance phase you recognize and acknowledge all of your emotions—anger, sadness, anxiety, abandonment. This is a time to share your feelings with others freely. Acceptance is the bridge that takes you beyond loss and separation into healing.

LETTING GO. This is a stage of forgiveness. You can begin to forgive yourself or others who may have hurt you. Here you let go of the past, begin to live in the present, and make plans for the future.

The Block to Recovery

Denying or resisting emotions that arise during the five stages of recovery will only prolong the journey to emotional well-being. You can block feelings of sadness and anger, but later they will return to haunt you, lingering for months or years. The following case is a good example of resistance and denial.

Ron, a man of 45, was divorced from his wife, Julie, five years ago. When the marriage ended both felt frustrated and bitter. Ron feels that the alimony Julie was awarded is outrageously high and that she is taking advantage of him. However, it's crucial to Ron that he continue to be able to act as a father to his three kids. So when Ron and Julie speak about arrangements for the children, Ron swallows his anger and maintains a polite and somewhat placating demeanor. Although five years have passed, Ron still feels angry when he thinks about his ex-wife. But since the consequences of expressing his anger could be potentially devastating, Ron instantly blocks out his anger with the fear that "the children will be taken from me." In some ways Ron is comfortable with staying fearful. By maintaining the fear that he will lose his children, Ron does not have to face feeling angry, rejected, abandoned and lonely. He can avoid looking at the cause of his failed relationship. Ron is stuck and unable to move ahead. He needs to learn from his mistakes and experience all the emotions generated by his separation.

All feelings are important and must be expressed, healed, and then released. Allowing yourself to feel the sorrow, hurt, loneliness, or anger that accompanies significant loss is not enjoyable, but it is a vital part of the recovery process. When you divert your attention, as Ron did, from the whole range of feelings generated by loss or separation to a single strong emotion (anger, anxiety, guilt, etc.), the many diverse feelings that loss and separation evoke will remain unacknowledged and often unfelt. The mind can maintain the illusion that only one feeling exists by:

1. Obsessively focusing on one aspect of the loss: the details of the actual event, some real or imagined injustice, something someone said, something you needed but didn't get, the ways in which your life is worse or better now, scary things that might happen in the future, and so on.
2. Developing a new situation in your life which continuously ties up most of your attention and energy: a serious problem, a new relationship, compulsive work activity, etc.

By generating the same thoughts or type of thoughts over and over, you can maintain the same emotion, causing this stage of recovery to repeat itself. This is called a repetitive thought pattern. It matters little whether the subject of obsession is real or imaginary. The important issue is how tenaciously you hold on to the thought pattern and the feeling it produces, whatever it may be. The following is a list of situations that can indicate obsessive focus on one emotion.

- The same scenes repeat themselves over and over again in your mind.
- You find yourself frequently thinking about what you should have said or done.
- After a great deal of time has passed, you still have made no attempt to replace your loss with new people, experiences, or things.
- You live a secluded life, interacting with few others. The intensity of your feeling leaves little room for other people.
- You enter a relationship immediately after a loss has occurred.
- You create one crisis situation after another so that a continuous feeling of panic replaces the unbearable feeling of loss.

All of these situations may be signs that deeper emotions associated with loss are being blocked or masked.

Releasing the Block

The following exercise will help you create affirmative statements to replace the repetitive thoughts that lock you into one predominant emotional response. These affirmations will be incorporated into the *Recovery from Loss Induction*. Using this exercise will allow you to have access to the feeling that you are blocking. Your resistance will decrease and you will be able to move to another stage of recovery. Do this exercise whenever you fell trapped or stuck by your repetitive thoughts.

There are two steps to this exercise. First, whenever you catch yourself repeating or reliving a situation over and over again, write down the thought connected to it. For instance, let's say the situation is that you have been fired from your job. The repetitive thought might be:

"I have just been fired. I'll never find another job."

Now, to replace the repetitive thought write down a statement that expressed your situation in a positive light. Concentrate on your strengths and the things that you can do. Acknowledge the existence of your emotions, but also the fact that your emotions will pass with time. When these guidelines are followed, the repetitive thought of "I've been fired. I'll never find another job," could turn into:

"I've been fired. But I found this job and I know I can find another. I can do it."

This positive thought is called an affirmation. Now, write down your repetitive thoughts and affirmations here:

REPETITIVE THOUGHTS: AFFIRMATIONS:

_____   _____

_____   _____

_____   _____

_____   _____

_____   _____

_____   _____

Next, make a copy of the affirmations you have written and post this list in a place where you can easily read it—your refrigerator, night table, or bathroom mirror. Review it at least twice a day—once in the morning and once in the evening. By keeping your affirmations in mind, you will be more likely to recognize repetitive thoughts when they occur. This will help you release the emotion you are holding on to and move on to another stage of recovery. Over time you may need to change certain affirmations. Some you will rewrite, some you will drop as you develop new affirmative statements.

The following is a list of general affirmative phrases which also may be helpful to you.

- I have the courage to live one day at a time.
- I can release the sorrow of my loss.
- I will enjoy life and appreciate the good things I have accomplished.
- I will create a new and promising life for myself.
- I can handle the difficult times. I will do it.
- I take care of my health and personal needs.
- I will make the right decisions and be responsible.
- I love myself.
- I will grow from my sorrow into a richer, stronger human being.
- I can do it. I can make it.
- My loss has given me tremendous insight and knowledge.

Programming for Recovery

As you practice the *Recovering from Loss and Separation Induction,* over time you will be able to:

Realize the truth of your circumstances and gain access to the full range of your emotions. Nothing you feel is insignificant or unimportant. The induction will help you to fully experience each emotion as it surfaces. You will become able to accept your emotions as being a natural part of your healing process.

Forgive all the people and things that you blame for your sadness and sorrow. The induction will enable you to let a feeling of compassion enter your mind, and "a greater kindness fill your heart."

Release the emotions that keep you tied to your loss and prevent you from recovering. You will become able to release the anger, sadness, and guilt that you have been feeling.

Heal. Healing takes place after you have gained access to your feelings, forgiven those involved in your loss, and released the emotions you have been clinging to.

The Total Induction

Now that you understand how the induction works, you are ready to use it. The *Recovery from Loss and Separation Induction* is used with the *Relaxation Induction* in Chapter 2. You may remember that the *Relaxation Induction* is divided into two parts. Insert the *Recovery from Loss and Separation Induction* between these two parts. The three components should not be separated from one another as they are used or taped—they should blend into one continuous flow. With this in mind, follow this procedure:

1. Turn to Chapter 2. Use the *Going Down Induction*.

2. Use the *Recovery from Loss and Separation Induction*.

3. Turn to Chapter 2. Use the *Coming Up Induction*.

Recovering from Loss and Separation Induction

Now, in your special place, allow yourself to reflect on the feelings that your loss (separation) brings up. Deep, deep, deep down inside yourself you know that [INSERT YOUR MOST HELPFUL AFFIRMATIONS HERE]. *Now, allow the emotions that are arising within you to pass right through you one by one. Watch them rise and pass. Feel each emotion as it rises and passes right through you. It can be sadness, or anger. It may be feeling abandoned or guilty. Just let any emotion surface and float to the top. You may be fearful of loss and your own sense of security, just let these emotions surface and float to the top. There is no need to resist, just let your body relax. Become aware of how your body is feeling. If you have any tension in any part of your neck or shoulders, let them relax. Now notice your breathing. Are your breaths short and shallow? If so, take a deep breath and relax your breathing, inhale in, and now, out.* [PAUSE AND WAIT 20 SECONDS, GIVE YOURSELF TIME TO INHALE AND EXHALE.] *Now, just relax your body even more, and continue to experience each emotion as it surfaces and rises to the top. Now allow your body and mind to accept them as being a natural part of your process. Let them flow into your awareness and let them flow out of your awareness, easily. No need to resist. Just let yourself flow with each and every emotion. And, as you drift into deeper relaxation, let yourself forgive all the things you have blamed. Forgive each person, forgive yourself, feel a compassion enter and flow through your mind. Feel a greater kindness fill your heart, and as you let go, let yourself feel more at peace, balanced, and more harmonious with life around you. Let go and release all of the anger and sadness you have been feeling. Let it go, just feel it pass, feel it flow through you and pass out of you, no need to resist. Just let it go, feel it pass out of you, and as you let these emotions go, feel a new sense of peace emerge. You know you are all right, you know you can make it, and you know you can do it. You know you have the courage to move ahead and beyond your loss. Now just begin to imagine yourself past your sorrow. It's behind you now. You may see yourself with friends or family, or you may see yourself alone in your special place. See yourself smiling, feeling at peace, feeling healthy and strong.* [PAUSE.] *Imagine yourself motivated once again, imagine yourself involved with activities that you enjoy.* [PAUSE.] *Your mind, body, and spirit heal each day. Each day you grow stronger, healing and recovering, healing and recovering. Feel yourself drift and float in a warm glow of healing thoughts and visions. Feel yourself float in a warm glow of healing energy, no need to resist, just drift and float. Now, just enjoy your special place, take your time, just enjoy your special place.*

What to Expect and Following Up

Use the induction once or twice a day for as long as you need it. Each individual will recover at his or her own pace. As you begin to feel better, continue to use the induction daily, keeping in mind that recovery is not linear. Some days you will feel great, you may even find yourself enjoying a day at the beach or lunch with friends, when all of a sudden a wave of sadness or anger could emerge from nowhere and engulf you. It will pass and you will feel fine again. This is a normal occurrence in separation recovery. When you feel you are past the critical emotional turmoil but still experience momentary strong emotions related to the loss, use the induction occasionally to help you reconnect with your inner sense of peace.

Case Study

When Edward's company transferred him to a different location some 400 miles away, he and Gwen were ecstatic. The transfer meant a promotion for Ed and the couple would finally be able to afford the house they had always wanted. They found the perfect home and within a month had fixed the place up so that it looked like they had lived there for years. Every day Ed went to work. He now had an office and a secretary. The guys at work were friendly and took Ed to the health club for daily workouts. Ed joined the company softball team. But most of the time Ed's thoughts were buried in his work. He had little time to notice much outside of the office.

Gwen's side of the story was much different. When she and Ed first moved into their house, most of her energy was spent gardening, and sewing, and generally fixing up the house. However, as time passed and there were fewer things that needed to be done, Gwen would go for hours at a time feeling lost and disoriented. Had she still lived in their old home, she would have visited one of her neighbors, or gone to the park, or visited the museum with her best friend, Liz. As the weeks dragged on Gwen began to feel more and more depressed. Pretty soon she was spending all of her time indoors watching television. She found it very irritating that Ed was never at a loss for things to do and had little free time to spend at home. The irritation eventually turned to anger, and when Ed came home at night he was met with a barrage of complaints and blaming attacks.

Gwen needed to realize that the restlessness and depression she felt was a natural reaction to the loss of her old home, neighbors, and friends. Since the new house and Ed's new job were things they both had always dreamed of having, Gwen thought that she should feel excited and was surprised and worried when the excitement was shortlived. She had left herself no room to feel the sorrow that leaving her hometown brought on. Since Ed was kept busy dealing with his new job, he was largely unaware of the separation reaction Gwen was having. Gwen saw his lack of attention as callousness and put all of her energy into feeling angry at Ed. This somehow seemed safer than admitting to the sadness she felt about the move.

Ed actually came up with the idea that Gwen should consult a hypnotherapist. By using the *Recovery from Loss and Separation Induction* twice a week for two months, Gwen became aware of her true emotions and of how she had blocked these emotions by staying focused on feeling angry at Ed. By the end of the two months, Gwen had done some mourning for her old life, met several new friends, and mostly let go of her resentment toward Ed.

Special Considerations

It is important to note that when you are going through your recovery process, it is easy to neglect your health and emotional needs. Should you experience any physical problems, see your doctor. Seek out as much emotional support as you can. Begin by talking with family and friends and, if needed, consider counseling to help you cope with your loss.

19

Surgery

For a moment just close your eyes and imagine your doctor saying, "You need surgery." Notice your physical and emotional response. Are your knees feeling a little weak? Is your stomach queasy? Do you feel a little light-headed? If you have ever had surgery, these feelings are familiar to you. Fear of the unknown, dying, separation from family and friends, and painful medical procedures are common concerns for those facing surgery.

The following cases illustrate the successful application of hypnosis before, during, and after surgery. They also show the emotional stress, fear, and anxiety that accompany surgery and anesthesia.

John was a volunteer in a hypnoanaesthesiology seminar. His four-hour surgery for prostate cancer was scheduled for the next day and he was eager to learn techniques for controlling pain, minimizing bleeding, and hastening recovery.

Throughout the seminar, several students worked with John to decrease his anxiety and fear. The instructor demonstrated pre- and posthypnotic suggestions for John's surgical procedure. At the seminar's conclusion, John reported feeling calm, positive, and empowered. His willingness to share his vulnerability and fears deeply touched the instructor and students alike.

Several days following the surgery John called the instructor to describe his experiences. He reported feeling no fear or anxiety whatsoever as he had gone into the operating room; instead he had felt prepared. A spinal block allowed him to stay awake throughout the procedure and he stated that he remained calm and confident the entire time. John used the hypnotic techniques learned at the seminar to minimize bleeding and discomfort. In the recovery room he experienced minimal pain. The doctors were pleased with John's speedy recovery and felt he would be discharged from the hospital ahead of schedule.

Susan was unhappy with her facial profile and had scheduled reconstructive surgery on her chin. Because she was allergic to the anesthetic medication, she chose to use hypnoanaesthesia. Prior to the surgery she attended four hypnosis sessions. With practice Susan mastered numbing the chin area, she would feel sensations of pressure but no pain during the actual surgery. During the operation she visualized a speedy recovery. One week after surgery Susan was observed to have minimal bruising or swelling from the procedure.

For liver and kidney transplants, the postsurgery recovery period is a precarious time during which the major concern is the acceptance of the new organ. To enhance and speed the acceptance of a new organ, a partnership between mind, body, and spirit is essential. Hypnosis can help in this process, as in the following case.

Three months after Greg's successful liver transplant his body was beginning to show signs of rejection. Although Greg had a strong will to live, he felt this new organ was not a part of him, but a stranger, an adversary. Hypnosis helped Greg accept his new organ and create a stronger partnership. During hypnosis sessions he visualized trusting his liver to be strong and healthy and imagined the medication as powerful and healing. Two years later Greg continues to stay healthy and enjoys hiking, writing music, and traveling with his band.

Hypnosis can be a powerful tool for surgical procedures in the preoperative, intra- (during surgery), and postoperative phases. For hospitalized patients with catastrophic illness, learning self-hypnosis can help surmount periods of private distress, help increase or regain autonomy, as well as motivate a patient to actively participate in his or her own recovery. Currently no study can identify an ideal time for hypnotic intervention. Ultimately the patient's individual needs will determine the best opportunity for hypnotherapy. Studies do show positive outcomes at any phase with the use of hypnotic intervention.

Here are some ways hypnosis assists patients before, during, and after surgery as well as throughout recovery:

- Prior to surgery, hypnosis can reduce anticipatory fear, anxiety, and tension, and increase confidence by developing a calmer, positive state of mind. A positive attitude will help a patient participate more fully in his or her health.

- Hypnotic analgesia can reduce or eliminate pain from illness and painful medical procedures prior to surgery.
- During surgery, hypnoanaesthesia can be used to replace or minimize side effects of anesthesia. The positive posthypnotic suggestions given before or during surgery can control bleeding, reduce the need for muscle relaxants, and increase postoperative pain control.
- After surgery, hypnosis can ease recovery from anesthesia, reduce or eliminate pain, nausea, vomiting, and bowel distress, as well as discomfort from other postoperative medical procedures.
- The recovery period may include healing from a wound or incision, regaining normal body weight, or increasing physical energy and psychological well-being—all of which can benefit from hypnosis.

When recovering from illness, disease, or surgery, the mind, body, and spirit connection plays an integral part in regaining health and well-being. Maintaining a positive attitude reduces stress and helps medical procedures to go more smoothly. This is not to say that worry, fear, and tension will just disappear with hypnosis; you may experience these emotions, as they are a natural response when faced with a pending stressful event. However, focusing on negative feelings can demoralize and depress you, inhibit your immune system, and slow healing and emotional recovery. Hypnosis will help keep your focus away from these negative feelings.

Prior to surgery, the simple *Relaxation Induction* can be given daily to reduce stress and tension. Another way to maintain a positive attitude is through the use of the *Rehearsal Induction,* which may go something like this:

Imagine yourself a few moments, or even a few hours, before surgery, whenever you choose. Begin to breathe easily, relaxing deeply, a pleasant calm flows over you, and as you relax more and more, you know you are being taken care of. You can just flow with deep relaxation, by the time you enter surgery you are completely relaxed. The surgeons are experts and are extremely capable, you are just fine, you are just fine. Now imagine you are in recovery and just opening your eyes, you feel relaxed, you are just fine, you feel comfortable and relaxed, all is well.

In Karl's case, a postsurgery rehearsal was given to encourage a positive attitude and enhance healing after surgery. Karl left his doctor's office with all the fears one can expect when given the news that he needed a quadruple bypass operation. Although the doctor assured Karl of a successful surgery, full recovery, and extension of life, Karl was frightened. He worried about losing his life, his family's distress, and a painful recovery. His doctor continued to promote a positive attitude by telling Karl, "As you regain your strength, and recover, you will be able to play golf again, perhaps better then ever."

Building on his doctor's positive suggestions, hypnotherapy was utilized to help Karl increase his confidence and reduce his anxiety. Prior to surgery, Karl's hypnotherapy treatment plan consisted of the *Stress Reduction Induction,* the *Healing and Recovery Induction,* and specific posthypnotic suggestions for a full recovery. The posthypnotic suggestion, or rehearsal, stated:

Imagine yourself a short time into the future, your successful surgery is behind you. You continue to regain your strength, each day you feel stronger, and stronger. Now just imagine getting back to your daily routine, see yourself enjoying your friends, see yourself on the golf course, see yourself teeing off, your swing is strong, you follow through, your body moves effortlessly, fluid movements. Just imagine enjoying your friends, your golf game, just see the entire game, see yourself playing a great game, you feel strong, energized. Each time you play, you regain strength and energy, you get better and better each time you play golf.

Along with hypnotherapy, Karl faithfully followed his doctor's advice, adhering to a health regimen that included medication, moderate exercise and a good diet. Karl continues to recover from his successful bypass operation. His health and energy are back; however, he still plays golf better in a trance than on the actual golf course.

A History of Hypnosis in Surgery

The use of hypnosis in surgery dates back to prechemical anesthetics, which were beginning to be discovered in 1846. The efficacy of hypnosis in surgery is supported by many studies, beginning with the first documented case in 1829 of a mastectomy performed by Jules Cloquet in France. This was followed by the work of English surgeon John Elliotson (1830), who performed many surgeries using hypnosis as the sole anesthetic.

In 1971, a treatment group of 15 open-heart surgery patients listened to audiotapes suggesting preoperativly systematic relaxation (Aiken and Hendricks). The treatment group had fewer negative psychological reactions, a shorter recovery period from anesthesia, fewer blood transfusions, and less hyperthermia than the control group.

Recent research reports success in the effectiveness of hypnosis with breech pregnancies. Eighty-one percent of the fetuses in an intervention group converted to vertex presentation. Other studies show that when hypnosis is used prior to surgery, it can reduce the the amount of anesthesia and muscle relaxants the patient needs; and soothing suggestions used during surgery may mean a quicker recovery. See Chapter 8 for more on childbirth.

Definition of Terms

Hypnoanaesthesia and Hypnoanalgesia are often used interchangeably because the difference between them is minimal.

Hypnoanaesthesia: Partial or total loss of sensation while in a trance state. Complete loss of the conscious experience of pain. In a hypnotic trance, the subconscious accepts suggestions equivalent to chemical anesthesia. Here is an example of posthypnotic suggestions in preparation for wrist surgery:

Imagine the pain in your wrist becoming less and less, all sensation leaving your wrist, your wrist becoming more and more numb, more and more numb, as if you had a shot of novocaine, or as if you had plunged your hand in ice cold water. Your entire hand is becoming more and more numb, right up to your wrist, becoming so very numb, your hand and wrist so numb, now, you may feel a slight sensation, and that's fine, the incision in your wrist may feel like the impression of a pencil being drawn across your wrist, or you may experience no sensation at all because your wrist is so numb, so very numb.

Hypnoanalgesia: Inability to feel pain while in a trance state by directing attention away from the pain. For example, while in the dentist's chair, just before minor dental surgery, Mark closes his eyes and imagines that he is lying on the beach in Hawaii. He focuses on the waves, the sand, the sun. . . . As the dentist begins, Mark feels no pain, yet he is fully conscious and awake.

Hypnoanaesthesia in Surgery

The use of hypnosis as the only method for anesthesia is not common for major surgery today. Chemical anesthesia is reliable and easier to administer. However, when a chemical anesthetic may be harmful, as in some cases of pregnancy, lung disease, and other medical conditions, hypnoanaesthesia can be an effective alternative.

Hypnoanaesthesia for Children

Children are especially receptive to hypnosis. Their trusting nature coupled with active imaginations make them good candidates for pre-

and postsurgery preparation. A child's world of make-believe can be used to strengthen the hypnotic suggestions. In 12-year-old Tony's case, he was exposed to meningitis and recommended for a spinal tap (lumbar puncture). Because Tony was allergic to local anesthetics, hypnosis became an appropriate alternative. On the day of the spinal tap, Tony's father performed the hypnotic induction just a few moments before the doctor administered the needle into Tony's lower back and continued speaking during the procedure. He began the induction:

Tony, think about relaxing your entire body, every muscle, relax all of the muscles in your back, right down to your lower back, just relax. Imagine you are sleepy and relaxed, imagine that you are beginning to dream, you dream about being a pilot, you are flying high above the ground, everything looks so small, so small. Soon you see the ground far away, the earth, mountains, flying so high, you look around the cockpit of your plane, it is just like the model you have at home, but now you are actually flying it, you are the pilot, you're in complete control. The dream becomes more and more real, you can see the blue sky, you can talk to ground control, they are saying everything is going great, you're doing a great job. You can fly anywhere you want, you can fly into space and back again, and now whenever you're ready you can land safely, be back on the ground feeling great.

Although Tony was aware of the spinal tap, he was unaware of any discomfort and became so involved in the induction that his father had to tell him when the procedure was completed.

There are many techniques for children of various ages. Young children are most responsive to storytelling to distract their attention away from the medical procedure.

Your Treatment Plan (Preparing for Surgery)

Five weeks of preparation are recommended prior to the date of surgery. This will give you plenty of time to utilize many hypnotic techniques. However, if you are scheduled for an immediate operation you can still benefit by choosing any of the inductions for surgery provided in this chapter. For the best results, follow the program in sequence with each exercise practiced daily. This list includes pre-, intra-, and post-surgery exercises.

Stress reduction. Maintain a relaxed, positive attitude by selecting the *Stress Reduction Induction* from Chapter 6.

Pain control techniques for surgical procedures. There are specific posthypnotic suggestions for pain control in medical procedures and surgery in this chapter. To enhance your program, use the additional pain control techniques in Chapter 10.

Healing Induction for Surgery. This induction preprograms your subconscious mind to be confident, secure, and relaxed while you are chemically anesthetized during surgery. The induction suggests, "Imagine yourself going into a deep healing sleep. Imagine a special healing place. As you drift into a soothing, healing sleep, all is in proper order, all is as it should be." The induction goes on to suggest "Your surgeon, anesthesiologist, nurse, and other medical professionals are highly competent, they watch you, protect you . . . As you awaken and regain total consciousness, you feel comfortable, relaxed, and you feel as if only a few moments have passed."

Postsurgery Induction. If you practice this induction prior to surgery, your subconscious will automatically activate the suggestions immediately after surgery. Recovery can be maximized by listening to an audio recording of the induction in postop.

There are three components to the *Postsurgery Induction*. First, anchor a comfortable, relaxed feeling to a cue word. The induction suggests, "Imagine a time when you felt the most comfortable, the most relaxed, and just keep this image in your mind for a moment. Now, cue and anchor this image and feeling by assigning a word or phrase to it, something that has a special meaning to you, like 'sunset, calm, blue, pink, or I am relaxed'." Next, the induction suggests a positive, and comfortable recovery from the anesthesia: "Imagine awakening, becoming more aware of your surroundings. The first thought that enters your consciousness is about how well everything has gone, I am fine, I am just fine." For the last component, controlling any physical sensations such as pain from the incision, nausea from the anesthesia, or any other discomfort from medical treatments, the suggestions are, "If you want to release any sensation, simply close your eyes, or focus on a stationary object in your room, perhaps the flowers on the dresser, or a picture on the wall. Now repeat your special cue word quietly in your mind. As you repeat your cue word, feel the comfort flow over you, warm and comfortable, the sensation becomes more and more comfortable."

Healing and Recovery Induction. The subconscious sees a picture in the mind and develops a blueprint for the appropriate behavior. For example, if you imagine biting into a lemon you will actually feel its tartness in your mouth; your subconscious reacts as if the lemon were real. The same is true when you visualize yourself recovering completely. Your subconscious sees the positive pictures and responds accordingly. Even if there is slow or partial recovery the positive suggestions and mental imagery given to the subconscious will still be powerfully effective. The *Healing and Recovery Induction* suggests, "Imagine yourself healing, imagine your wound or incision healing so quickly, healing and recovering so quickly, so fast, your doctors are amazed and pleased." This induction continues to reinforce the healing process, suggesting, "Imagine yourself fully recovered, imagine yourself energized, strong, and vibrant." The induction concludes with a mental blueprint for life beyond recovery, "See yourself back to your normal routine, at work, see yourself productive and energized, or see yourself with friends or relatives, you are enjoying yourself." Surgery is rarely a pleasant experience, but, in retrospect you may gain some valuable insight that will enhance your life. The induction suggests, "As you recover, you have gained new insight, and appreciate life. You may not know the answer yet, and that's fine, it will become more clear to you as you recover more and more each day."

Taping the Total Induction

You may choose to record all of the pre- and postsurgery inductions or just the one that fits your need. Once you have chosen the appropriate induction, follow these steps to tape your total induction:

1. Turn to Chapter 2. Use the *Going Down Induction.*

2. Use the *Healing Induction for Surgery* or select the specific induction that fits your need from the *Treating Specific Procedures* section later in this chapter.

3. Record the *Coming Up Induction* from Chapter 2

Healing Induction for Surgery

As you relax deeper and deeper, just imagine yourself going into a deep healing sleep, a deep healing sleep. Imagine a special healing place, it could be by the ocean, in a temple, or any place that you want. As you drift into a soothing, healing sleep, you give in to the most restful sleep you have ever experienced, and as you drift into healing sleep, you sleep sound, deep, and restful, and as you sleep all is in proper order, all is as it should be. Your surgeon, nurse, anesthesiologist, and other medical professionals are highly competent, they are in charge and take great care of you, they watch you, protect you, there is nothing for you to do but simply relax, you are being cared for, all is as it should be, all is as it should be. During your procedure, your Inner Observer, Guide, or God is watching and protecting you. Your power for healing is activated and regulates your body every step of the way, every moment that passes your subconscious is activated for instantaneous healing, every procedure moves along easily and effortlessly. Upon successfully completing your procedure, you continue to heal, you heal very quickly now and when you awaken from your healing sleep you feel comfortable, you feel good, and you feel as if only a few moments have passed. As you awaken and regain total consciousness, you feel comfortable, relaxed, and you feel as if only a few moments have passed.

Postsurgery Induction

As you relax deeper and deeper, imagine a time when you felt the most comfortable, the most relaxed, remember a time when your body felt relaxed and free from any discomfort, your body moving easily, just think of the most comfortable time, remember how you felt, you felt relaxed, at ease, just keep that image in your mind for a moment, let it linger, as you recall the image, you can even feel the comfort and relaxation. Now, cue and anchor this image by assigning a word or phrase to it, something that has a special meaning to you, like, "sunset, calm, blue, pink, rose, or I am relaxed." Now quietly, in your mind, repeat it several times, much like a mantra. As you repeat it over and over quietly in your mind, you feel the comfort and relaxation that your special word represents. From now on, whenever you want to feel this level of comfort, just say your special cue word [INSERT CUE WORD] and feel the comfort immediately. Continue to relax deeper and deeper and now imagine yourself slowly beginning to awaken from your surgical procedure, as you relax deeper and deeper imagine awakening more and more, becoming more aware of your surroundings. The first thought that enters your consciousness is about how well everything has gone, how well everything has gone, you are fine, you are just fine. It feels as if only a few moments have passed, it feels as if only a few moments have passed, as you awaken more and more you feel comfortable, relaxed, comfortable, relaxed, so very comfortable, so relaxed, you take a few comfortable breaths of air returning to full consciousness. You begin to notice your surroundings, more and more, you become aware of your body and how you feel, you are comfortable and you are relaxed. You may feel nothing at all, just total comfort, or you may have a slight sensation. You may want to keep the sensation or you may want to let it go, if you choose to release it, simply close your eyes or focus on a stationary object in your room, perhaps the flowers on the dresser, or a picture on the wall. Just focus on a pleasant object and at the same time repeat your special cue word [INSERT CUE WORD] slowly, over and over in your mind, at the same time, focusing on the flowers in your room, or the picture on the wall, or gently close and relax your eyes, and as you repeat your cue word, feel the comfort flow over you, gently, easily, warm, and comfortable, light, warm, and comfortable. Imagine the sensation, first a little tingling, then a little warmth, or a little coolness, whatever is comfortable for you, the sensation becomes more and more comfortable, more and more comfortable. Feel the comfortable sensation flow through your body, cooling, or warming, feeling more and more comfortable, feeling more and more comfortable. This pleasant sensation spreads through and around your entire body. As you return to full consciousness this area feels comfortable and you feel relaxed, you feel good.

Healing and Recovery Induction

As you relax deeper and deeper, imagine yourself healing, imagine your wound or incision healing so quickly, healing and recovering so quickly, so fast, your physicians are amazed and pleased. Imagine the area of your surgery healing right before your eyes, your skin healing, becoming normal healthy skin, smooth and pink and healthy, mentally travel down your body, visualize every cell in your body regaining strength, your blood count is good, every bone in your body healthy and strong, every muscle in your body gaining strength and elasticity, every organ working at maximum efficiency, your heart rate relaxed and strong. Imagine yourself gaining strength everyday, getting stronger and stronger. Imagine yourself fully recovered, imagine yourself doing something that you enjoy, see yourself energized, strong, vibrant, you are joyful, enthusiastic about life, your body is loose and comfortable, you may want to see yourself running along a long stretch of beach, or walking along a country road, just imagine life in the most positive way, in your mind's eye see yourself back to your normal routine, at work, see yourself productive and energized, or see yourself with friends or relatives, you are enjoying yourself, laughing, engaged in conversation, as you recover more and more you begin to see some positive aspects about your surgery, perhaps you have gained new insight, and appreciate life a little more. You continue to recover more and more each day. Just imagine your blueprint for total health and well-being. Each and every day you continue to heal and recover and reach your goal of total health and well-being.

Treating Specific Procedures

Follow the guidelines provided in the *Taping the Total Induction* section in this chapter to personalize and record the posthypnotic suggestions for specific medical procedures.

Intravenous Therapy. An IV is administered to all surgery patients. This procedure is the most effective way to route medication or anesthesia to the circulatory system. Initial discomfort from the needle or the burning sensation of the medication going through the veins can be reduced or eliminated. Depending upon the location of the IV, you will insert "arm" or "hand" into the induction, as indicated below.

Relax your neck and shoulders, breathe gently into your neck and shoulders, feel the relaxation in your neck and shoulders, now feel the relaxation travel down your arms, down your arms, your arms becoming heavy, so heavy, so filled with relaxation, all the way down to your fingertips. Now focus on the arm (or hand) that is not receiving the IV, and now begin to imagine a layer of cushion, like a thick pin cushion covering the soft tissue and veins of your arm (or hand), remember you are focusing on the arm (or hand) that is not receiving the IV, imagine the pin cushion becoming thicker and thicker, it rises above your arm (or hand), above your skin and veins. As you focus on this arm (or hand), the exact same thing is happening to the other arm (or hand), however you continue to concentrate on this arm (or hand), your other arm (or hand) experiences the same, or 100 times more, 100 times more, now, just imagine, imagine a small pin pricking the pin cushion, the cushion is soft and pliable, and because it sits on top of your skin, you feel nothing at all, you may feel the pressure of the pin cushion against your skin, and that's fine, you may feel the pressure of the pin cushion, and that's fine, as you imagine the protective pin cushion on your arm (or hand), you may be surprised that, all along, your arm (or hand) receiving the IV feels nothing at all, it too, feels as if it had a very large pin cushion protecting it, you may even feel the same small amount of pressure, or you may be surprised that the IV has been gently inserted, the procedure is completed, and you feel relaxed, and comfortable.

Blood Draws. Blood is drawn for analysis in many medical treatments. A blood draw may be repeated several times, causing pain from the needle puncture. The objective here is to numb the area of the skin receiving the needle puncture and allow the blood being drawn to flow easily. Repeat this paragraph at least three times or until it is effective.

Imagine your special place, far away from any concerns, all is well, you are being cared for, you can take some time out for a mini vacation. Imagine that special place, see it in detail, see all aspects of your special place, now really relax into it. In this special place, imagine the alcohol being gently rubbed on your skin, feels cold, like an ice cube, numbing the skin, numbing the skin, feels so cold, just like ice, numbing the skin, you may not even be aware that blood is now being drawn, you allow your blood sample to flow easily, you know it is a small amount, you can easily let it flow. Now as soon as you have finished, your blood clots properly and the puncture heals quickly, it is a simple procedure that you can do many times, because you are able to numb your skin, you are able to let a blood sample flow easily from your veins, and you are able to heal quickly.

Dressing Changes. Recovering in postop may include changing the dressing of a wound and protecting it from infection. The goal here is to be relaxed and infection-free during the procedure and during healing.

Now just relax, focus your attention on your incision. As you focus directly on it you may feel some sensation, and that's all right. Begin to imagine the sensation as a coolness, feel a cool and comfortable sensation in and around your incision, as this comfortable coolness increases, it soothes your wound, the coolness reduces swelling and inflammation, feel it soothing, and healing. Imagine what color coolness might be, imagine a cool, soothing color, now imagine this cool, soothing color surround and flow through your wound, healing, keeping your incision clean, cool, healing, and now each and every time the dressing of your wound is replaced, all you have to do is imagine the coolness and the color of the coolness surrounding your wound, surrounding the incision, the coolness keeps this area comfortable, and relaxed, comfortable and relaxed, and now just imagine your wound completely healed, the skin is healthy, the incision is clean and completely healed, the skin is pink and healthy, completely healed, the skin is pink and healthy.

Removing Stitches. The sensation of having your stitches removed can be uncomfortable. Again, the objective is to be relaxed and pain-free during this procedure.

Relax, deeper and deeper, your wound has healed. It is healthy and healed, it is so healthy in fact that the stitches that have been holding the tissue together are no longer needed. Now that makes you happy, and because you have healed so well, you no longer need these stitches, you are now looking forward to removing them, you are now ready to let them go. Focus on the stitches, imagine them shrinking in size, shrinking, become thinner, thinner, smaller, imagine them shrinking in size, perhaps to the size of a strand of hair, so small, so slight, and as they are removed, it feels like a small strand of hair being gently pulled through your fingertips, as if you are running your fingers through your hair, and the strands of hair flow through your fingers, gently flowing. Just imagine your stitches gently flowing, out of your skin, gently flowing out of your skin, and just imagine them all removed, your skin is healthy, your skin is healthy and healed.

Spinal Tap. Lumbar puncture is a diagnostic test performed to obtain a fluid called cerebrospinal fluid or CFS, which bathes the brain and the spinal cord. The procedure requires a needle to be inserted into the spine to obtain the spinal fluid, and although a local anesthetic is most often used, it can be a painful experience. The objective here is to reduce trauma, discomfort, and pain.

Relax with every breath you inhale and exhale, breathe in and out, relax more and more. Now begin to let your mind wander to a place and activity far away, begin to play with your imagination and imagine yourself far away, imagine that your body is resting and is comfortable, you body position is comfortable, your body is loose and relaxed, the muscles in your back are loose and relaxed. Your body is becoming so comfortable, so heavy, so relaxed, so comfortable, it feels so heavy, and as your body grows heavier, your subconscious feels lighter and lighter. Now focus on your breathing, notice only your breathing. Relax, focus on your breathing, breathe easily, effortlessly, breathe in and breathe out, now simply notice your breathing, notice how it moves into your nostrils, down into your lungs, notice exhaling. Exhale all of your breath, remember to let this action be easy and effortless, exhale, just notice your breath and nothing else for a moment, notice, as you inhale, notice the air moving into your nostrils, down into your lungs, breathing so easily. Now exhale, relaxing as you exhale and inhale, simply notice your breathing. Become less and less aware of your breathing as you let your mind wander, becoming less and less aware of your body as you let it relax. Just feel a warm and comfortable relaxation envelop you, becoming less and less aware of your body. Now just let your mind wander, wander far away, far away from your body, far away, now just imagine yourself completely engrossed in a specific activity, [INSERT SPECIFIC ACTIVITY HERE] *it may be an athletic activity like skiing, or playing a game of tennis, or it may be an artistic activity like painting, or it can be an activity like problem solving, like a science project. Now, just let your mind focus on this activity and become engrossed in this activity, see it in as much detail as you can, imagine every aspect of this activity, imagine telling some one about it, explaining every detail of it. Now just imagine yourself so completely engrossed, so completely absorbed. You can be completely involved for as long as you want, you can stay in your special place for as long as you want.*

What to Expect and Following Up

If you are scheduled for surgery, the daily use of the *Relaxation Induction* will help prevent presurgery stress. To include all aspects of the surgical procedure (before, during, after, and recovery), begin practicing as soon as possible. Practicing the inductions five weeks before surgery should give you enough time to become comfortable. If time is limited, you can still greatly benefit by using the *Relaxation Induction* along with the specific induction that is right for you. By using the inductions daily, the surgery and medical procedures will go more smoothly, tension, stress, and pain will be reduced; you will also have a quicker recovery.

Feeling more energized and having a sense of peace and wholeness, you can return to your daily routine. In the recovery phase, use the *Healing and Recovery Induction* daily for a week and as you progress, cut back and use it only as needed, until you no longer require the reinforcement for healing.

Special Consideration

Designing your total health plan for surgery requires several considerations—your commitment, self-knowledge, and motivation. To fully understand your condition and medical procedures, ask your physician specifically what to expect in the pre- and postoperative phase. Inform your physician, surgeon, or other health care providers about your hypnotherapy program. Patients in surgery can now request soft music to be played during surgery, or even a taped induction if head phones can be used. Many nurses and doctors are proficient in hypnosis and can also assist you. To enhance and strengthen your program, you may want to seek the help of a professional Hypnotherapist who is a certified Hypnoanesthesiologist, or a certified Medical Hypnotherapist.

Professional Associations

The associations listed below can refer you to qualified Hypnoanesthesiologists and Medical Hypnotherapists in your area.

National Board for Hypnotherapy and Hypnotic Anesthesiology
6037 West Baniff Lane, Ste. A
Glendale, AZ 85306

American Association of Professional Hypnotherapists
P.O.Box 29
Boones Mill, VA 24065

The Palo Alto School of Hypntherapy
The California Institute for Medical Hypnosis
2443 Ash St. Ste. D
Palo Alto, CA 94306
(800)774-9766

20

Overcoming Depression

When Gabrielle contracted mononucleosis, she was bedridden for four weeks. Accustomed to leading an active life, she was now unable to work, go out with her friends, or attend her daily dance classes, among other things. Some days even showering was a chore for her. When she finally regained her strength, she no longer wanted to do any of the things she had done before. She found herself sleeping all day, not eating, and avoiding phone calls from friends, relatives, and co-workers. Even though the sickness had passed, the depression that came along with it lingered.

According to the National Institute of Mental Health, more than seventeen million people in the United States experience depression each year. Research shows that men, women, and children are all affected by depression, although women experience it at roughly twice the rate of men. Specific biological, life cycle, and psychosocial factors may contribute to women's depression. However, age, lifestyle, and environment are added stresses for all people who suffer from depression.

Distinguishing Minor Depression from Major Depression

Depression is more than just a bad mood. Some symptoms of minor depression include loss of energy, motivation, and appetite; despite these symptoms, however, those suffering from minor depression are still able to function normally and get necessary things done.

When depression pervades every aspect of life, when getting out of bed to go to work becomes a problem every day, the depression is no longer minor. According to the *Diagnostic and Statistical Manual of Mental Disorders*, a major depression exhibits at least five of the following nine symptoms, and these symptoms must have been present for at least two weeks:

1. Depressed mood most of the day, nearly every day
2. Diminished interest or pleasure in almost all activities of the day, nearly every day
3. Significant weight gain or loss when not dieting, and decreased appetite nearly every day
4. Insomnia or hypersomnia (sleeping too much) nearly every day
5. Abnormal restlessness or a drop in physical activity nearly every day
6. Fatigue or loss of energy nearly every day
7. Feelings of worthlessness or excessive or inappropriate guilt nearly every day
8. Diminished ability to think, concentrate, or make decisions nearly every day
9. Recurrent thoughts of death, or suicidal thoughts or attempts

(Adapted from *The Depression Workbook*)

Severe depression can be serious and life threatening and should be treated immediately. If you are having thoughts of suicide, call your local suicide prevention hotline or your doctor—get help now. Regardless of how bad you may be feeling, depression can be treated successfully.

Depression is a dark filter that clouds your ability to discern reality from fantasy. You begin to believe your fatalist future visions, such as "No one will ever love me again," "I'll never find another job," or "My life will never be the same." Regardless of the origin of depression, one thing is certain: negative, self-defeating thoughts perpetuate it.

The journey out of depression does not have to be long or even difficult. This chapter will provide you with simple and effective hypnotic exercises for feeling good again. The hypnotic inductions and techniques will focus on eliminating or reducing negative thinking that can contribute to depression. You will also master the skill of *manifestation*, increasing positive feelings and working towards positive goals, to create a more joyful life beyond depression.

Working Towards Positive Goals

Before you examine your options and choices for treating your depression, jump ahead to the intended outcome of your treatment plan. Review the following goals and make a mental note of the ones that are most important to you. Return to these goals again later in the process.

- To enjoy a good night's sleep and awaken feeling refreshed, ready to meet the challenge of the day
- To feel hopeful and view the future in a positive way
- To feel relaxed, calm, and productive
- To take pleasure in your usual activities, like baking, jogging, or working in the yard
- To have a healthy appetite and be at a comfortable weight
- To feel healthy and strong
- To feel more confident and proud of your accomplishments
- To be focused and able to concentrate and make decisions
- To experience your full range of emotions in a productive way

Facts About Depression

The symptoms of depression are emotional, physical, and psychological and can be experienced individually or simultaneously. In order to understand the dynamics of depression, here are some common facts.

Triggers

Although researchers are getting closer to understanding depression, no one knows exactly what happens in the brain to cause it. We do know that most major depression involves an imbalance of chemical messengers, or neurotransmitters, and the limbic system, which regulates emotions, appetite, sleep, hormone levels, and behavior. Neurotransmitters are part of a delicately balanced communication network that controls the limbic system. When these chemicals are in balance, you feel good; when the balance is disrupted, you feel depressed. Here are some specific triggers that can disrupt this balance:

Stress. It is normal to feel sad, angry, or depressed during stressful periods that occur because of the death of a loved one, loss of income, or divorce. But chronic stress can develop into depression.

Traumatic events, such as an abusive childhood or an injury may lead to depression.

Genetic factors and personality types. Depression may run in the family. Low self-esteem and lack of confidence are factors that can cause or increase depression.

Specific diseases or major illnesses. Immune system diseases, illnesses, surgery, and physical pain can cause depression, as in Gabrielle's case.

Medications. Certain medications have side effects that can cause depression; consult with your physician if this is an issue.

Alcohol or drug abuse can cause an imbalance of brain chemistry leading to depression.

Hormonal imbalance. Changes in hormone levels may contribute to depression. A fluctuation or a decrease in hormones during childbirth or menopause can precipitate depression in women. Postpartum depression is fairly common among new mothers; approximately 80 percent of new mothers experience stress-related symptoms of depression.

Chronic patterns of negative thinking. What you think affects your brain chemistry. Constantly focusing on the painful, disappointing parts of life can have a lasting detrimental impact on your brain chemistry and your moods.

Negative thinking

While constant negative thinking, such as self-blame or inadequacy, can fuel the fire of depression by adversely affecting the chemical balance in your brain, the converse can be true as well—a chemical imbalance can intensify negative thinking. Finding a way out of this cycle may seem impossible, but changing your pattern of thinking can lead the way.

Once you understand how your thought processes work, you can begin taking steps to change the patterns of negative thinking that cause or intensify depression.

Negative thoughts are myths you have accepted about yourself, your family, or your life as truth, based on information accumulated throughout your lifetime. For nearly every topic or experience, you may have painful memories, judgements about yourself, even labels like "stupid, incompetent, or worthless."

For example, John is never satisfied with any of his achievements, no matter what he has accomplished. He believes that he is not good enough and he doesn't try hard enough; these thoughts produce anxiety and depression. John measures himself by past experiences with his father, who set high standards for his children yet rarely praised them for their good work.

Chronic negative thinking in your conscious or subconscious mind can become a habitual thought pattern. When these silent, or not so silent, thoughts are triggered, you may first notice an emotion instead of the thought. For example, when Laura arrived at work one morning, she noticed that she was suddenly upset. When she examined her emotions, she realized that she was scheduled to complete a task that she had struggled with in the past. She was dreading the day's work because she already believed that she would fail. Every time she started to work, she was interrupted by the thought, "I can't do this. I already know that I am not good at this." Her perception of the situation not only made her upset, but prevented her from trying to do her work.

Principles for Change: Recognition, Realization, and Refuting Negative Thoughts

Recognition. The moment you notice a drop in mood, a mood swing, or a thought that is negative, stop, take a deep breath, and recognize the thought process. You may find that you have been engaged in this process for the last ten minutes or more. Simply by recognizing the thought process itself, you will have stopped its progression.

    Realization. In the past, you have accepted all negative thoughts as truth. Stop doing this. Do not give value to these thoughts because they do not tell the truth about who you are; they only lead you into depression. There is far more to you and your experiences than these negative thoughts. But these depressing thought patterns tend to filter out all the positive things to appreciate about yourself.

    Refuting negative thoughts. Once you recognize a negative thought, refocus your attention on refuting the negative messages your thoughts are trying to sell you. Look for the balancing positive experiences in your life; remember your strengths and accomplishments. Think about the things that nurture you, things that you genuinely enjoy.

    When you apply these three basic principles, you will be able to gain a more realistic view of events and situations.

Setting Up Your New Plan

There are two major inductions for recovering from depression. The first, the *Overcoming Depression Induction,* is designed to incorporate the principles for change—recognition, realization, and refuting negative thoughts. The *Manifestation Induction* will assist you in focusing on positive goals and increasing your positive feelings. Together these two inductions will help you meet the following objectives:

- To change your negative thought process
- To incorporate new responses into your life
- To become a happier, calmer, and healthier person

- To create a positive future
- To bring joy into daily living
- To feel good again

Programming for Results

The *Overcoming Depression Induction* is designed to replace the habitual negative and self-defeating thoughts that cause or increase your depression. The posthypnotic suggestions reprogram your subconscious to accept positive alternatives to negative thinking.

Your subconscious as protector. Your negative thoughts and thought patterns have become habitual. The *Overcoming Depression Induction* will break those habits by suggesting: "Your subconscious is your protector, and, as your protector it will alert you to negative thinking. The moment you recognize your negative thought process in progress, you immediately stop and take a deep breath."

Principles for change. At this time the induction reinforces the principles for change by suggesting: "Realize your negative thoughts have no value. They cannot solve a problem, nor make you feel better. They have no value."

Reprogramming for positive goals. The induction concludes with the positive goals set forth in the beginning of this chapter. The induction suggests: "Imagine a checklist of positive goals, the list may include enjoying a good night's sleep, awakening feeling refreshed in the morning, feeling hopeful, feeling productive, and taking pleasure in leisure activities . . ."

The *Manifestation Induction* is designed to help you master a positive process of thinking and reprogram your subconscious. Manifestation is the ability to take an active role in creating what you want— what you want the "here and now" to be like, what you want the "future" to be like, and how you want to feel about it.

Building trust and confidence in the future. The way to build this trust is to create a positive future place in your mind. The induction suggests that you "project yourself a little into the future. . . . Imagine a future place, a place of serenity and peace."

Inserting your positive goals. Here, the induction gives you the opportunity to insert your new positive goals: "Now, create your future, imagine that you have achieved your goals, imagine what they look like, imagine every detail."

Reinforcing the positive goals. Positive emotions help to make a goal achievable. The induction suggests: "Add to this future image positive feelings. Add joy, happiness, imagine yourself smiling."

Accepting joy and happiness. It may be difficult for you to accept feeling happy and joyful. You may feel that you don't deserve to be happy when other people are suffering. The induction removes these apprehensions by suggesting: "Your manifestation serves a positive purpose in life. Imagine your manifestation benefits everyone."

Bringing the future into the present. In order to feel that your goals are achievable, you must bring them into your present realm. The induction continues: "Now bring this manifestation to the present, bring the images, feelings, and goals to present time. You own these positive feelings, they have been inside of you all along, and all you need to do to bring them forward is to create the space, allowing yourself to experience joy, happiness, peace, and serenity."

Allow for flexibility. "Be careful what you wish for" is a popular adage and needs consideration here. Just in case your manifestation is not in your best interest, allow for flexibility. For example, in concentrating on achieving career success, you may fail to recognize the effect it may have on your family and psychological well-being. Working late and concentrating only on success may in the long run not be what you were hoping for. Let your manifestation take a shape that will serve your highest good. The induction suggests: "Know that your manifestation is being created for you in the most positive way. As your manifestation develops, it may not look the same as you imagined. It will be better than you imagined. You will recognize your manifestation coming to pass by how you feel; each and every day you feel better and better."

Designing Your Total Induction

You are now ready to put your total induction together, combining each component into one continuous flow. To do so, follow this procedure:

1. Turn to Chapter 2. Use the *Going Down Induction*.

2. Select the *Overcoming Depression Induction* or the *Manifestation Induction* that follows.

3. Turn to Chapter 2 and use the *Coming Up Induction*.

Overcoming Depression Induction

Relax more and more, and as you drift deeper into relaxation, let your thoughts relax. Relax your thought process, nothing to think about right now, just imagine yourself in a peaceful, special place and because your mind and thoughts are in a resting place, your subconscious mind becomes open to positive posthypnotic suggestions. Your subconscious is your protector, and, as your protector it will alert you to negative thinking. The moment you recognize your negative thought process in progress, you immediately stop, take a deep breath, and realize your negative thoughts have no value. They cannot solve a problem, nor make you feel better. They have no value, they have no value, they have no value, these thoughts only give you negative messages about yourself, let them go. Remember you are a valuable person, you are loved and cared for, you are smart and creative. Now, just relax more and more, notice your breath, just notice your breathing, and refocus your awareness on your breathing and relax deeper, now refocus your thoughts and imagine positive goals, achieving positive and healthy goals, imagine a checklist of positive goals. The list may include enjoying a good night's sleep, awakening refreshed in the morning, feeling hopeful and positive about the future, feeling relaxed and calm, feeling healthy and strong, feeling productive, and taking pleasure in leisure activities, like seeing friends, taking a walk, going to the movies. Each new day you feel more confident, you have positive goals for the future and you make good decisions daily, you take care of your health and well-being, you experience joy, happiness, and laughter, you embrace the good times as well as the bad times, and treat yourself with compassion and understanding, you allow friends and family to support you, and you feel better and better every day, better and better every day.

Manifestation Induction

And now just relax deeper and deeper, from this quiet place of deep relaxation I would like you to project yourself a little into the future, it may be tomorrow, or the next day or next month, or you may see yourself six months from now, not too far into the future, just a little into the near future. As you project yourself into the future, imagine the easy flow forward, gentle, easy, no need to rush, just an easy flow forward, let your subconscious choose the future time, imagine a future place, imagine a future place, a place of serenity and peace, just imagine it for a moment, a place of serenity and peace, linger here, all is as it should be, allow yourself to relax and simply feel peaceful. Now, create your future, imagine that you have achieved your goal, imagine what it looks like, imagine every detail, (pause, and give yourself all the time that you need, when you are ready to continue, do so) there is no need to know how you achieved your goal, just imagine the end result in the most positive way. Now, add to this future image by placing positive feelings. Add joy, happiness, imagine yourself smiling, imagine yourself dancing with joy, or running, jumping, laughing, really feel those positive feelings now, remember the last time you experienced a good belly laugh, your whole body felt it, you laughed, feeling the full force of joy, now, if you are not experiencing total joy, that's all right, as you practice this manifestation you will experience the positive feelings more and more each time you practice this manifestation. Just create your future manifestation in the most positive way, each time you see it, add a little more detail, each time you see it, add more positive feelings. I would like you now to add the final portion to your manifestation, imagine your manifestation to serve a positive purpose in life, imagine your manifestation benefits everyone. Your manifestation brings joy and happiness to you, and to everyone. Now, bring this manifestation to the present, bring the images, feelings and goals to present time, you own these positive feelings, they have been inside of you all along, and all you need to do to bring them forward is to create the space, allowing yourself to experience joy, happiness, peace, and serenity. Your manifestation is being created for you right now, just let it go, know that your manifestation is being created for you in the most positive way. As your manifestation develops it may not look the same as you imagined. It will be better than you imagined, you will recognize your manifestation coming to pass, by how you feel, each and every day, you feel better and better each and every day, you feel more alive, motivated, joyful and happy, each day your manifestation is being created, each time you imagine your manifestation it grows stronger and stronger, you are surprised at how much lighter you feel, how at peace you feel, you let each day unfold, flowing easily with change, flowing easily with life, better and better every day, now just relax for another moment, enjoying the place you are in.

What to Expect and Following Up

You may choose either the *Overcoming Depression Induction* or the *Manifestation Induction.* Use the induction you have chosen and listen to it daily for one month. You may alternate inductions or listen to them both regularly, as any combination is appropriate. You should notice an improvement in your mood in the first few weeks. As you progress you may want to reduce your use to weekly reinforcement sessions.

Refer to other inductions in this book that will support and speed your recovery from depression. Some recommended ones are: *Stress Reduction Induction, Sleep Induction, Self-Esteem Induction,* and *Motivation Induction.*

Case Study

One evening Dee experienced unusual pain in her abdomen accompanied by back pain and a severe headache. She was rushed to the hospital for immediate medical treatment. In the emergency room, the internal bleeding was stopped and her condition stabilized but, unfortunately, Dee experienced a miscarriage and lost partial vision in one eye. During her first month of recovery, her brother died in a fatal motorcycle accident. This additional loss increased Dee's depression. She felt hopeless and anxiously anticipated the next tragedy. She no longer found any joy in life. Even though Dee's physical health returned (she adjusted to her limited vision and returned to a normal routine) she was depressed. Dee received support from many sources, including family, friends, and a therapist. But despite her abundance of resources, Dee could not stop her negative thoughts and the depression they caused. Eventually she sought help through hypnosis.

Her hypnotherapy treatment plan involved setting positive goals. She wanted to (1) regain her confidence and self esteem; (2) reduce stress; (3) stop her continual loop of negative thinking; and (4) reprogram a new image of herself as being empowered and in charge of her life.

Dee used the *Overcoming Depression Induction* for the first week. Her thinking became more positive; she began making plans, seeing friends, and smiling more often. The following week she incorporated the *Manifestation Induction* and after the third week she alternated the inductions daily. By the end of her first month of hypnotherapy, she felt "back to her old self" and was positive about the future.

Special Considerations

In addition to using the inductions, there are other important steps that should be taken. At the first sign of depression, or the recurrence of depression, talk with a friend or family member. Consider any medication or change in prescription that may be adding to your low mood. Explore other possibilities such as a change in diet, seasonal changes, or lack of exercise. If your depression lingers for more then two weeks or if you're feeling suicidal, experiencing physical ailments such as nausea, intestinal irritability, or insomnia, see your doctor. Your overall plan for overcoming depression may combine counseling, medication, and hypnotherapy, for complete healing.

21

For the Hypnotherapist: Special Considerations

It is possible to be an effective therapist, to achieve continued and consistent success with psychotherapy, and yet not be an effective *hypno*therapist. If, for example, you come to hypnotherapy with unrealistic expectations of the influence it can have and the changes it can bring about, you may strive to exceed the reasonable limitations of the hypnotic experience. A hypnotherapist who believes that anything and everything is possible may become overly ambitious. In the process, he will seek to exert boundless influence. The goal of the hypnotic induction then becomes compliance, with the hypnotherapist's motives distorted by a quest for personal aggrandizement.

At the opposite end of this spectrum is the skeptic. If a professional engages in the practice of hypnosis with a high degree of reservation and suspicion about the value of hypnotic treatment, he will not project a positive attitude or be able to function with true conviction.

Regardless of whether the hypnotherapist has either too much confidence or too little, the relationship with the client will be weak— possibly even doomed before it begins.

There are some desirable characteristics for a hypnotherapist to have that will contribute positively to the hypnotic experience. An effective hypnotherapist will:

1. Encounter each client as a unique individual whose problems should not be quickly categorized.
2. Have the ability to identify problem areas, assess their severity, and determine the type and scope of the induction that is to be used for treatment.
3. Be perceptive of the client's emotional needs.
4. Maintain an objective view of the hypnotic experience.
5. Keep personal problems or aspirations from distorting the treatment.
6. Accept and deal with emotional displays that arise during treatment.

Setting Up Your Environment

Your practice may be in your home, office, or clinic, or you may meet your client in his home, hospital room, or garden. Regardless of the location, you will need to eliminate outside interference as much as possible. The space that you create around yourself and your client should be exceptionally calming and relaxing.

The relaxed atmosphere. Soft colors, comfortable furnishings, lush green plants, and soothing music contribute to a sense of restfulness and calm.

Troubleshooting locations. If you are going to work in a location other than your office or home, you will need to familiarize yourself with the area. Check for any potential causes of disturbance. Ask if there is a telephone nearby that could ring and disturb your induction. Find out if children are usually playing outside, or if construction is going on in the neighborhood. Prior to your appointment, make a list of the possible disruptions, then seek to circumvent them before you engage in a session with your client. Take the phone off the hook, arrange for someone to watch the children for an hour or two, or schedule your appointment when the construction crew is having lunch or finished for the day.

Coping with external disturbances beyond your control. You can't stop the roofers from repairing the roof, the telephone from ringing in the next office, dogs from barking, or the jackhammer from blasting away outside the window. However, you can use these sounds to your advantage by incorporating them into your induction. If you are dealing with the rhythmic sound of the jackhammer or the roofers' hammers, you can suggest to your client, "The constant rhythmic sound you hear will drive you deeper and deeper into relaxation." If the source of the disturbance is airplanes departing or arriving at the airport, you could suggest, "The roar of the motor, its drone, signals you to let relaxation hum through your body, relaxing you, relaxing you deeply." If children are playing or the telephone is ringing, you could suggest, "Be aware of all the normal sounds around you, they are unimportant to this session, place them out of your awareness, and from now on whatever you hear will help you relax more deeply."

Your appearance. Remember that how one person looks and acts can greatly influence how another person feels. For example, you are sitting in the waiting room of your dentist's office. The woman across from you begins to yawn. You watch her as she yawns again, and in just a few minutes you are yawning too.

You are standing in line at the bank. The man ahead of you is dressed to the nines. His sparkling white starched shirt is buttoned to the top, and his handsome necktie is bound tightly and efficiently around his neck. He keeps running his fingers around the collar as if to loosen it. As he keeps tugging, he seems uncomfortable. Soon you are tugging at your own collar, regardless of the fact that you are wearing a T-shirt.

Similarly, you influence your client by the way you act and look. If you wear an expensive dark suit, dress shoes, and a silk blouse or designer shirt, and your client is dressed rather casually, he or she will probably feel subordinate and slightly self-conscious. If you dress comfortably—neat, but casual—your client will be put at ease. Visual appearance will not take any attention away from the purpose of the session.

The hypnotic induction begins at the door. You should convey a sense of comfort and peace the moment you greet your client. Your client may be nervous and unsure of what to expect, or he may have just gotten off work and rushed to your office and be fearful of being late. If your client arrives in an apprehensive mood, anxious or tense, you need to transfer your positive feelings and relax your client. If you speak in a well-modulated, calm voice, and move surely but quietly, you will be projecting the message that "everything is under control here. I am peaceful. Things will move calmly." By relaxing your client the moment you meet him, you will have begun a relaxation process that will lay the groundwork for the actual induction.

The Initial Interview

During the interview or first consultation, you will gather information concerning the client's problem. The more fully you understand the causes of a problem, the better you will be able to define it and resolve it.

At the same time, it is also necessary to educate your client about hypnosis. The more the client understands, the more confidence he will have in the hypnotic process. This is also the time to establish rapport and trust. By reassuring your client of his safety, he will be receptive to a good working relationship.

Listening for the Motivation

After your client states the reason he wants to use hypnosis (to lose weight, to reduce stress, to stop smoking) you need to listen to determine what your client's incentive is for solving the problem. By questioning and listening discriminately, you can select the strongest motivational factor and incorporate it into the hypnotic induction. In the following interview, listen for the motivation for change.

Joanne, a legal aid attorney, has just stated that her reason for seeking the help of a hypnotherapist is to stop smoking.

Hypnotherapist: Why do you want to stop smoking, Joanne?
Joanne: Well, I guess for my husband's sake. He hates it.
Hypnotherapist: Are there any other reasons?
Joanne: Well, I know it isn't healthy and I'm beginning to cough quite a lot.
Hypnotherapist: I see. Now is there any other reason that comes to mind?
Joanne: Well, to be honest with you, I have a brand new baby granddaughter. My oldest daughter brings the baby over on weekends. I don't want to smoke around her. I don't want her to see me smoke — I don't even want her in a room where someone is smoking.

In this case, Joanne's greatest motivation is her granddaughter. Joanne's hypnotic induction will be designed to include her major reason to stop smoking. The *Nonsmoking Induction* in Chapter 5 will be used, and the emphasis on her granddaughter will be incorporated into the induction. The suggestion would sound something like this: "Just imagine yourself holding your granddaughter, you are both breathing clean, fresh air and she sees you as a nonsmoker. You are being a good role model. It feels wonderful to be such a positive influence on her."

Defining the Problem

During the first interview, allow sufficient time to define the problem. Discover the causes by asking when, where, with whom, and under what conditions a symptom occurs. During the interview with Joanne, you discover that she rarely smokes at home. However, she chain-smokes at work, because she is under tremendous stress. This indicates she needs to reduce her stress reaction at work in order to reduce her addiction to cigarettes. The interview continues:

Hypnotherapist: How much do you smoke, Joanne?

Joanne: Oh, I guess it's about two packs a day.

Hypnotherapist: Where do you smoke most often? Is it after meals, at home, at work, as you commute, while you watch TV?

Joanne: Let's see, I don't smoke at home in the morning and I don't smoke in my car. I do like to have a cigarette after meals, but at work I'm a chain smoker. I'm under a lot of pressure, and smoking helps me to relax.

Now you have the when, where, and why of Joanne's smoking habit. She smokes *when* she is under stress. She smokes at work (*where*), and she smokes to relax at work (*why*).

Pinpointing Problems and Finding Alternatives

New patterns can be established much more easily if old ones can be replaced by functional alternatives. Joanne needs new alternatives to smoking at work. She decides to take a few minutes for a break and to relax by taking a walk, if only in the hallway of her office building. Alternatives were discovered as follows:

Hypnotherapist: If you were under stress and you decided not to have a cigarette, what would be the next best thing that would relax you? Remember, it can't be a job or another duty to perform. You can't think, "Well, I won't smoke, so I'd better clean out my desk drawer"—unless cleaning out a drawer relaxes you.

Joanne: I know that if I could go for a walk during my break I would feel more relaxed.

Hypnotherapist: In your hypnotic induction, you will include new options, new behaviors to replace old behavior patterns. Going for a walk will be your new option. The *Nonsmoking Induction* will suggest, "When you feel stressed, you will go for a walk. You can walk outside your office building or just in the hallways of your building. You will walk away from your desk, away from pressure." You smoke when what you need is relaxation and comfort. When you need to relax and feel assured, what else could you do?

Joanne: Talk to Nancy for a couple of minutes, or get some reassurance from somewhere, let off steam.

Hypnotherapist: Who is Nancy?

Joanne: A woman who works in my department.

Hypnotherapist: Your new option, then, can be to talk to Nancy. Also, what about going to a quiet place, the ladies lounge, your car, or a room that is not used by others, and taking a minute or two to review the positive aspects of your life, to mentally list your capabilities, and plan something you can look forward to?

The hypnotherapist and Joanne have worked together to determine some alternative patterns of behavior that will be acceptable. Joanne has also been made familiar with the relaxation technique so that she can call upon it when she needs it.

The Induction

On completion of the interview, your client should feel relaxed, confident, and eager to begin. You have gathered information and know what suggestions to give.

Before introducing the inductions, make sure your subject is in a comfortable position. You may instruct him at this point to close his eyes. If a person sits with legs and arms crossed, or completely upright as if in a straight-backed chair, there is little hope of him achieving the relaxation necessary for a successful induction. Encourage your client to stretch out or lean back into a soft chair as the induction proceeds.

Your voice is important—your tone, rhythm, and the special delivery techniques that can be incorporated to achieve specific goals.

As explained in Chapter 2, your basic voice should be either *monotone* or *rhythmic*. The monotone is a drone without inflection or variety in pitch or rhythm. The rhythmic voice rocks or lulls the subect into relaxation through the use of speech that has an anticipated stress pattern: "*You* are going *deep*er, *deep*er, *deep*er into *total* relax*a*tion."

For emphasis and reinforcement, you may use word distortion, such as "feel those muscles become *loooose* and relaxed." You may use raised pitch for posthypnotic suggestion or to give the command to come up from an induction. You will be able to maintain an uninterrupted rhythm by using connective words, and you may insert silent pauses when time is needed for your subject to respond to a suggestion such as "Now tighten your right foot."

The induction can vary in length from a few moments to 25 or 40 minutes. It depends on your technique.

As your subject relaxes, some physical signs to indicate the depth of the trance will occur. Some of these signs include:

1. *Paling of the face* as the blood circulation slows. This indicates that the subject is in a state of relaxation.
2. *Shallow breathing*, which indicates that your subject is entering a deeper trance state. Initially, your subject may breathe at a regular pace. Then a deep sigh occurs and the breathing becomes more relaxed. Breathing becomes so slow and undetectable that some subjects report feeling as if their breathing had stopped.

3. *Muscles relax* in the face, the jaw slackens, and the body becomes very still.
4. *Muscle catalepsy* may occur. This is a rigidity of certain muscles. The muscles become taut and immobilized. The "paralysis" exhibited is really the subject's interpretation of how he or she would be if actually paralyzed; that is, the rigidity is not induced by the motor nerves. The action is behavioral rather than physiological. Twitching fingers or rapid eyelid movement may also occur. (The eyelid movement should not be confused with rapid eye movement [REM] in the sleep state.)
5. *Physical responses to your suggestions* may be evident. If you describe an enjoyable place where the subject can play, have fun, smile, and be joyous, look for a smile on his face. If you suggest that a subject's arms are so heavy they can't be lifted and you then instruct the subject to try to lift them, watch the arms struggle against an invisible force. As your client visualizes and reacts to simple suggestions, you will know that he is in a responsive trance and ready to accept further suggestions.

Depending on the type of induction you use, you may request that your subject describe something to you or carry on a conversation with you during an induction. The subject's speech under hypnosis will often be slurred, slow, and show little inflection, as if the person were talking in his sleep. If a subject is talking with careful attention to language, he has probably not progressed beyond a light trance state.

Coming Out of the Induction

When you have concluded the induction and are ready to bring your subject back to full consciousness, alter your voice, changing the tone from soothing to conversational and alert. Your subject should begin to move around, and eyes should open upon the suggestion given in the *Coming Up Induction* in Chapter 2. Be sure to include suggestions that will produce good feelings, such as "feeling refreshed," "wide awake," "alert," or "feeling wonderful." Color in the face should return in a few moments. Give the client a short time to recover, and watch for signs of drowsiness.

Spend a few moments discussing the experience: how the client felt during the trance state, how hypnosis contrasts with a conscious state, and how the client feels now. If he is still a bit dazed, spend additional time talking with him, give him a soft drink or cup of coffee, and make sure he is fully awake before he leaves.

When Relaxation Turns to Sleep

In most cases, a subject's eyes will open when the command is given to "Open your eyes and return to full consciousness." However, sometimes a subject will fall asleep during the induction. You can bring the subject back by altering your voice, making it louder and more direct.

In a situation such as this, it may be difficult to know if your subject has accepted the suggestions. If he has actually blocked out everything and just enjoyed a nap, he may have missed certain suggestions. It is a good idea to record the induction on a cassette tape, give it to him to listen to at a later date, and instruct him to assume a less comfortable posture or to sit in a straight chair so that he is not prone to fall asleep.

Audrey immediately fell asleep each time her nonsmoking induction was given. As soon as her eyes closed she was asleep, and soon after she was snoring. Yet when she returned to the hypnotherapist's office after several weeks of this routine, she was a nonsmoker. One can only assume that even in her deep trance state she was able to accept suggestion.

Sometimes a subject will sleep in order to prolong the comfortable feeling of the trance state. It is a form of escape and not a cause for alarm. If the subject does not respond to the command, "Now you will come back from your sleep, back to full consciousness, now when I count to ten you will be fully awake," you may simply allow the person to continue the nap and awaken when he feels the need to.

Exercising Discrimination

There are specific problem areas for which hypnosis is not well-suited, and there are certain types of clients you should not attempt to treat. (This latter recommendation is not directed at the highly-skilled, qualified professional who has extensive experience; it is aimed, instead, at the hypnotherapist whose background in severe mental and emotional disorders is not extensive.)

When you are in doubt about the acceptability of a client, it would be wise for you to recommend the client to another therapist, an agency, or outpatient clinic. The following three types of clients are generally candidates for referral; the individual whose expectations regarding hypnosis are completely unrealistic, the borderline personality, and the psychotic.

The person who has unrealistic expectations. This is a client who would otherwise be an appropriate subject for treatment, but who has the view that hypnosis is a magic cure-all. A patient such as this may seek hypnosis as a form of treatment because he has already undergone a series of unsuccessful therapies. He is looking for something quick and easy. Even though hypnosis often works more rapidly than other forms of treatment, it cannot be expected to accomplish the impossible. For example, you could not expect to induce revulsion where passion is in great evidence; that is, you could not successfully use hypnosis to eliminate strong feelings a client had for a friend, relative, or lover.

Alene, a florist in her mid-40s, had a history of broken romances with men, all of whom shared similar characteristics and habits. Her relationships were full of emotional turmoil and always terminated rather quickly—the longest one having a duration of four months. At one point in her life, she became involved with Alan, who was charming, successful, romantic, and a sensitive sexual partner. However, Alene had to share Alan with several other women because he responded enthusiastically to most of the available women he met.

Alene was jealous and sought hypnosis to relieve her misery. She requested an induction that would create total amnesia in regard to Alan. She wanted to be inducted into the "deepest trance" and made to forget Alan's existence—even his name.

The hypnotherapist explained that any suggestion to forget Alan would be ineffective. Even if by chance Alene was able to experience "Alan amnesia," the condition would only be temporary, and the next time she saw him the relationship would resume where it was before her hypnosis.

It was suggested that Alene undergo psychotherapy to investigate the reasons for her behavior and to discover why she subjected herself repeatedly to the same type of individual. After doing this groundwork, she was able to use hypnosis to increase her self-esteem. Once her feelings about herself improved, she became more discriminating and, if she did not meet anyone she found suitable, was not afraid to be without a male partner.

The borderline personality. This is a person who may have bouts of deep depression, feel victimized, and have simultaneous fears of engulfment and abandonment.

A person who is a borderline often cannot endure or experience the anxieties that will accompany the exploration of his problem. This individual may not acknowledge the magnitude of his problem or understand that the problem's source is not compartmentalized and self-contained, but reaches out into several behavioral areas.

Often, too, the borderline individual may be receiving many invisible benefits from his symptoms; so many, in fact, that he has reached a level of comfort with his *dis*comfort. The need for the benefits he derives from the neurosis may win out when he attempts to battle the neurosis itself.

The psychotic is a person suffering from severe thought or mood disorders. As stated before, hypnotherapy can be used with all types of people with mental and emotional disorders, but it is imperative that the hypnotherapist be a skilled professional with a wealth of experience. Many hypnotherapists may not have the training and technique necessary to combat problems that may arise.

Prepsychotic and psychotic subjects may react with any of a variety of intense emotions: rage, uncontrolled crying, screaming. They may have tics, speech problems, lack of physical coordination, localized tenderness, or sensory disturbances. Some people may experience hallucinations, amnesia, and erotic fantasies and impulses.

Hypnosis used as the *sole* treatment of severe disorders may either intensify the existing condition, or have no effect at all. However, hypnosis cannot create or bring about a psychotic episode where no precondition exists.

Dealing with Fearful Subjects

If you have a subject who becomes fearful or reports feeling uncomfortable, you can suggest, "You know you can always return from an induction because you are in full control. You may choose whether you wish to continue the induction or return to a fully conscious state and discuss your fears and discomfort." If the subject chooses to return to full consciousness, you will discuss the unpleasant feelings, focusing on one at a time.

Sometimes when a subject comes up from an induction he complains of a headache or some slight disturbance. In this case, you should hypnotize the subject again, using the *Relaxation Induction,* and suggest that the individual will "feel refreshed," "full of energy," and "wonderful," upon coming up and coming back. But even without rehypnosis, the subject's symptoms will disappear within a short period of time after he has come out of the trance state.

22

For the Hypnotherapist: Special Techniques

Age Regression

When an *Age Regression Induction* is used, it permits the subject to go back in time to review earlier surroundings and incidents in his life. For example, if you asked a 50-year-old to return to the first house or apartment he ever lived in, he would quite likely be able to describe each room, the surrounding neighborhood, and to name his playmates who lived nearby. He could tell you about events that were important to him at that time. These would be ones which produced some strong emotion, such as fear, joy, pride, or anger.

Studies have recorded some startling results obtained through age regression. Subjects who were given intelligence tests at various chronological age levels performed on the test in accordance with the age to which they had been regressed. For example, a subject who was regressed to the age of eight passed the test which was at that same level of intelligence measurement. He could not take a test at the next level and perform successfully.

Erika Fromm reported the case of a 26-year-old Japanese American who was born in California. The man stated that he did not know any

Japanese and could not speak it; however, when regressed to levels below the age of four he spoke Japanese easily.

Regression is often used in hypnotherapy to recover a past traumatic situation. After a problem has been traced to its source, it is easier to determine in which areas treatment is needed. During the induction, a subject may relive a scene in an immediate way (as if he were a participant at a regressed age level) or he may view the past event from his present perspective.

In Chapter 7 on treating phobias there is a short discussion about using the *Age Regression Induction.* The induction in that chapter is designed especially to uncover the source of an abnormal fear. This same induction can, however, be adapted for use in other problem areas — any area in which the source of the original trauma is sought. It is recommended that the subject who wants to try regression during self-hypnosis first seek counseling with a psychologist.

What follows here is a procedure to be used by the professional as he employs age regression techniques with a subject.

Getting permission. After the subject has achieved a state of relaxation through the *Relaxation Induction,* direct the subject to ask his subconscious for permission to trace the development of the problem, to go back to the original trauma. Suggest to the subject:

> *You can find out if it is safe for you and valuable for you to learn the cause of the problem. You will ask your subconscious and you will get a signal that tells us that we should or shouldn't go back to the scene that set the stage for your problem. If it's OK to enter the past to learn more about the problem, let yourself take a deep breath.*

Using ideomotor finger signals. Next, have the subject determine the fingers to be used for responses from his subconscious. The subject will decide which fingers will signal which responses. Four responses will be necessary: "yes," "no," "I don't know," "I don't want to answer." Say to the subject:

> *When you have become completely relaxed, focus your attention on your fingers. Repeat the word yes . . . yes . . . yes . . . over and over until you notice which finger is your "yes" finger. Keep thinking the word yes, and soon you will notice a little tug or twitch or sensation in one of your ten fingers — that will be your "yes" finger.*

When the subject's finger moves, reinforce the choice by saying, "Yes, your right index finger is your 'yes' finger." Then say:

> *Now repeat the word no over and over, while watching for any sensation, twitch or movement in another finger. That will be your "no" finger.*

When you notice that your subject is moving another finger, again acknowledge his choice by saying, "I see your left index finger is your 'no' finger." Repeat this procedure, directing the subject to select an "I don't know" finger and an "I don't want to answer" finger.

Now that you have established the ideomotor finger signals, you are ready to ask some preliminary questions. These questions help the client orient back to the traumatic scene without eliciting any specific memories. Here's an example of a therapist's questions and the client's responses.

Is there anything that happened to you in the past that set the stage for your fear? [YES.] *Is it something that happened before you were 18?* [YES.] *Before you were ten?* [YES.] *Before you were five?* [NO.] *When you were six?* [NO.] *Seven?* [YES.] *Were you at school?* [NO.] *Were you at home?* [YES.] *Was it after school?* [YES.] *At night?* [YES.] *Were you alone?* [I DON'T KNOW.] *Do you think your father was home?* [YES.]

When you have established certain facts about the trauma, then explain:

I want you to go back in time, to the scene that set the stage for your problem. As you go back in time, your subconscious will do the work. The subconscious will go through your memory as if it were a file box. You don't have to think or remember; your subconscious can do all the work. If you see a troubling experience from the past, don't try to relive it. Look back on it from the present time. Look back as if you were seeing a movie. Just keep going back, back, back to the scene that set the stage for your problem. When your subconscious can see the scene that set the stage for your problem, your "yes" finger will rise.

Repeat these suggestions for several minutes. If no "yes" signal is given, try this alternative approach. Tell the client that he or she is working too hard at remembering the past.

Your subconscious will do all the work. I want to tell you a story that you might enjoy. And while you are listening, your subconscious will still be working, looking further and further into the past. But you can relax and listen to the story. And when your subconscious knows the scene that set the stage for your problem, your "yes" finger will rise.

You can now keep the conscious mind busy by describing a train trip, a long hike in the forest, or the road leading to your grandfather's cabin. Whatever story you choose should be a long sequence of minute events and observations:

You know how it is on a train. The porter holds your elbow as you step up into the car. There's steam rising from pipes by the

> *tracks. You pull your suitcase up the stairs and start down the aisle. You put your suitcase in the overhead rack, you take a seat just as the train lurches and begins to move. Someone on the platform waves. Children are running alongside as the train gathers speed . . .*

Keep telling the story until you see the "yes" finger rise. Periodically during the story, remind the client that the subconscious is doing all the work and in a while the "yes" finger will signal that the scene has been found.

Viewing the original trauma. When the client signals that he or she is aware of the traumatic scene, give the following suggestion:

> *In a moment I'm going to ask you to go through that scene, the scene that set the stage for your problem. You'll see the whole scene, as if it were a movie, from start to finish. You'll see the whole scene unfold. You'll see the action, you'll hear what is said. As you start the scene, you will signal by raising your "yes" finger. And when you have finished the scene, when you have watched and heard everything, your "yes" finger will rise again. Now go ahead and start the scene. You can signal that you are starting the scene by raising your "yes" finger.*

The client has now mentally reviewed the traumatic event. Ask the client if it's all right to share with you the scene he or she has just witnessed. If there is a "yes" signal, give this suggestion:

> *In a moment, I'm going to count to three. When I count to three you can tell me what you saw and what you heard. When I count to three you can begin to describe the scene to me. You can talk, you can say what you saw and heard when I count to three.*

The client will now describe the scene using a thick, lazy voice. You can ask simple, direct questions, and, in most cases, the client will answer them. Reassure the client as the information surfaces.

> *Of course, as a child, you* [felt afraid and ran . . . did the best you could . . . had moments of cruelty like all children . . . felt angry at your father], *but those hurtful days are over. You are grown up now. The cord is cut to those painful days. The cord is cut and you are fully grown. You did the best you could then, but you are stronger and wiser now. Stronger and wiser. You can accept that those days are past. The cord is cut. You are grown up, so much stronger and wiser.*

Be sure at the end of the induction to always ask the fingers if it's OK for the client to remember the traumatic scene. Otherwise, suggest that the scene will remain forgotten until he or she is stronger and ready to know.

Pair Bonding and Anchoring

Pair bonding is a method used to associate a pleasant emotion with an undesirable behavior or unpleasant experience. For example, Carol was allergic to dust, but usually reacted only if she saw that her environment was dusty. Then she began to cough and have all the symptoms of an asthma attack.

Carol was asked to tell about a time when she was outside enjoying fresh air and breathing freely with no difficulty. Carol then recounted an experience she had when she traveled on the Oregon coast. She got up every morning just before dawn and walked on the beach while the sun was coming up. Those mornings had remained as some of the most pleasant in her life, having occurred at a time when she felt energetic and in perfect health.

The hypnotherapist used Carol's positive experience and the pleasant emotions that it elicited to eliminate Carol's undesirable reaction to dust. During the induction the following suggestion was made:

Imagine yourself walking along the shore on the Oregon coast, breathing clean, fresh air, the sun is just coming up and you are breathing clean, fresh air, feeling wonderful, breathing easily. From now on, whenever you notice dust anywhere, you will recall immediately the clean, fresh air of the ocean and you will breathe easily, freely again.

Carol was required to go back in time to a pleasant scene, one which had an element (in this case, fresh ocean air) that was in direct opposition to the element that caused the problem (dust-filled air). In pair bonding, you must first identify the negative element that is the major contributor to the person's problem. Then you can "match" that problem to some experience that will counteract it.

For example, consider this problem: A young man is afraid of telling his parents about his work and his lifestyle because he expects disapproval. He has become mentally alienated from his parents. The negative element is his fear of lack of approval.

Now the task is to identify an element that would be in direct opposition to disapproval, and the answer is, of course, approval. The young man is then asked to tell you about a time when he felt distinct approval. Next, during the induction, the subject regresses to the time of approval and relates the whole incident.

He describes the scene. He is at the high school science fair with his parents. They are walking down the long rows of tables looking for his project. As they approach his display, which details the major functions of the brain, they see a ribbon pinned to his project. He gets closer, reads the ribbon, and sees that he has won first prize. At the same moment, his father also realizes that it is first prize and a look of pride sweeps over his face. He reaches out and touches his son on the right shoulder, pats him, and pulls him over into an awkward sideways hug. Later, he hears his father telling his grandparents about the award. His father was bragging about him and saying that it was the best project in the fair.

You suggest to the young man that the gesture he will use to signify approval will be a tap on his right shoulder. He will use this as a cue to reexperience the approval he felt at the science fair. Thus, the bond is made between the positive emotion and any future experience in which he may anticipate disapproval. As he begins to reveal information or important feelings to his parents, feelings that he had previously felt would bring him disapproval, he now taps himself once on the right shoulder to elicit the positive emotion.

This type of bonding or anchoring can be productive in changing behavior, particularly in eliminating fears. The subject can regress to a time when he or she was healthy, loved, enthusiastic, or popular. A variety of physical gestures can be used to trigger the feeling evoked by the positive experience. To remember joy, you might turn your ring around to recover the emotional experience of the day you became engaged. You may put one hand in the other to trigger the positive experience of walking hand in hand with your mother in the country — a time when you felt loved. Any number of past positive experiences can be used to alleviate the negative emotions that accompany a given negative experience (taking a plane, crossing a bridge, going on a date, speaking in public).

Using Imagery and Language Patterns

The rehearsal. Prior to an induction, a rehearsal of the scene you will use during the induction can reinforce the images. For example, before you begin the induction, ask your subject to describe a perfect situation that relates to his area of interest, the problem area for which he is using hypnotherapy.

Bob, a baseball player, described his perfect situation this way:

I walk right up to the plate and get in position. My energy is high. I am excited but clearly focused. I know I am going to hit a home run. I see the pitch, feel myself concentrating as the ball approaches. I get a perfect hit. The ball seems to sail out of sight, to disappear. My feet fly around the bases effortlessly and when I come across home plate my teammates' uniforms are a blur of green and white jostling up and down as they congratulate me. My whole body is high and I feel as if *I* have won the game. I am ecstatic.

Now this positive description can be used in Bob's *Improving Your Athletic Performance Induction*. Bob will imagine playing baseball with the same feelings, emotions, and concentration he had in the above scene.

Using the appropriate vocabulary. Using the correct terminology, the vocabulary that best fits the subject's experience, can make the imagery more believable to your subject. For example, instead of telling a golfer "You are going to hit the ball off the small wooden peg stuck in the ground," it would be better to say "You are in the perfect position to tee off. You enter your back swing and execute your motion perfectly." To a dancer, you would suggest, "You see yourself in position, ready to begin your pirouette . . . " To a tennis player you would suggest, "As you return the serve back across the court, you can feel the ball hit the sweet part of your racket."

Listening to the subject's language. As your subject talks to you, be aware of his language patterns, of the kind of images he uses during ordinary conversation.

Among the various types of language patterns you might easily notice are: (1) Use of short, declarative sentences. ("I am at the top of the class. But now I can't study. Everything distracts me. I'm going to flunk out.") (2) Use of sentences that often end with an uplifting inflection, as if the speaker were asking a question or seeking approval. ("You see, I was walking down the street? And I saw my father coming toward me?") (3) Use of long, rambling sentences. ("It seems that when I go to see her she is always, well sometimes, she is not there very long or she says she has to go or something, but I don't know, so I tell her . . . ") (4) Use of strong harsh words or phrases ("fed up," "freaking out," "wiped him out," "cut me down"). (5) Use of muted, subtle language that veils emotion. ("My family does not care for those whose experiences are more limited than theirs.")

If you recognize a definite language pattern as your subject speaks, you may enhance the effectiveness of the induction by incorporating that pattern into the induction. For example, if you noticed that a subject was using the pattern described in item 5 above—the subtle language—you would not want to use phrases that were overly strong or blatant. If you had a subject who used the harsh expressions described in item 4, you could incorporate colloquial speech into the induction.

You will also notice that as people speak, they use imagery that falls into one of three categories: visual, auditory, or kinesthetic. Auditory images include such things as "the rain *pounding* on the roof," "the lonely dog *howling* in the yard," "the computer *clicking* and *whirring* away." Of course the visual images refer to what you see: "the three hills blurring on the horizon," "the farmland looking like the rich dark squares of a mammoth cake," "the open manhole like a large mouth exhaling smoke."

Kinesthetic experiences include "the feel of brick under your feet,"

290 Hypnosis for Change

"silk against your skin," "the sun on your face," or the "buoyant sensation of floating on water."

Some people tend to use more of one type of image than another. For example, would the following sentence groups be representative of someone whose imagery was predominantly visual, auditory, or kinesthetic? See if you can identify each group with one type of imagery.

1. My roommate was really cold to me.
   The exam was a pushover.
   I came out just riding high.
   I think the attorney wanted to sway the jury.
   The prosecutor was just trying to keep afloat.

2. When I talked to him on the phone, he was short with me.
   He was shining when he was onstage.
   The words he spoke were beautiful.
   I left the movie in an ugly mood.

3. His mind is buzzing with new ideas.
   That name really rings a bell.
   The headlines just screamed at me.
   The democratic headquarters hummed with excitement.

In group 1, the words *cold, pushover, riding, sway,* and *afloat* all relate to touch or physical sensation. The prevailing mode here is kinesthetic.

In group 2, the clue words are *short, shining, beautiful,* and *ugly.* The person is predominantly visual.

The sentences in group 3 represent a person whose orientation is auditory.

Now that you can identify each type, you may wonder what purpose your awareness will serve. Your perception about a subject's use of imagery can be helpful as you put together a "tailor-made" induction. By using similar language and reinforcing the induction with certain kinds of images, you are making sure the subject can relate to the induction and feel an affinity for it. The more appropriate the induction is for each subject, the more successful the individual's experience will be.

Bibliography

Books

Birkinshaw, Elsye. 1981. *Think Slim—Be Slim*. Santa Barbara: Woodbridge Press.

Blakemore, Colin. 1977. *Mechanics of the Mind*. Cambridge: Cambridge University Press.

Burns, David D. 1981. *Feeling Good, the New Mood Therapy*. New York: New American Library.

Carlson, Richard. 1992. *You Can Be Happy No Matter What*. San Rafael, CA: New World Library.

Carlson, Richard. 1993. *You Can Feel Good Again*. New York: Penguin Books, Inc.

Cleve, Jay. 1996. *Out of The Blues*. The Berkeley Publishing Group.

Coates, Thomas J., and Thoreson, Carl E. 1977. *How To Sleep Better*. Englewood Cliffs, NJ: Prentice-Hall.

Cooke, Charles Edward, and Van Vogt, A.E. 1965. *The Hypnotism Handbook*. Alhambra, CA: Borden Publishing Company.

Copeland, Mary Ellen. 1992. *The Depression Workbook*. Oakland, CA: New Harbinger Publications, Inc.

Cousins, Norman. 1979. *Anatomy of an Illness as Perceived by the Patient*. New York: Bantam Books.

Crasilneck, Harold B., and Hall, James A. 1985. *Clinical Hypnosis: Principles and Applications, Second Edition*. Orlando, FL: Grune & Stratton, Inc.

Davis, Adelle. 1954. *Let's Eat Right To Keep Fit*. New York: Harcourt, Brace, and World.

Davis, Martha; Eshelman, Elizabeth Robbins; and McKay, Matthew. 1995. *The Relaxation & Stress Reduction Workbook, Fourth Edition*. Oakland, CA: New Harbinger Publications, Inc.

Edson, Lee. 1975. *How We Learn*. New York: Time-Life Books.

Edwards, David D. 1978. *How To Be More Creative*. Mountain View, CA: Occasional Productions.

Ewy, Donna and Roger. 1970. *Preparation for Childbirth*. Colorado: Pruett Publishing Co.

Fanning, Patrick. 1988. *Visualization for Change*. Oakland, CA: New Harbinger Publications, Inc.

Feldenkrais, Moshe. 1972. *Awareness Through Movement*. New York: Harper and Row.

Fieve, Ronald R. 1981. *Moodswing*. New York: Bantam Books.

Fromm, Erika, and Shor, Ronald E. 1979. *Hypnosis: Developments in Research and New Perspectives*. New York: Aldine Publishing Company.

Gagne, Robert M. 1965. *The Conditions of Learning*. New York: Holt, Rinehart, and Winston.

Gawain, Shakti. 1978. *Creative Visualization*. Mill Valley, California: Whatever Publishing Co.

Ghiselin, Brewster, ed. 1954. *The Creative Process*. Berkeley and Los Angeles: University of California Press.

Haley, Jay. 1973. *Uncommon Therapy*. New York: Ballantine Books.

Hall, John F. 1961. *Psychology of Motivation*. New York: J.B. Lippincott Company.

Harner, Michael. 1980. *The Way of the Shaman*. New York: Harper and Row.

Henderson, Charles E. 1983. *You Can Do It With Self Hypnosis*. Englewood Cliffs, NJ: Prentice-Hall.

Hilgard, Ernest R. 1977. *Divided Consciousness: Multiple Controls in Human Thought and Action*. New York: John Wiley & Sons.

Hilgard, Ernest R. and Josephine R. 1994. *Hypnosis in the Relief of Pain*. New York: Brunner/Mazel.

Kent, Fraser. 1977. *Nothing To Fear*. Garden City, NY: Doubleday & Co.

Kroger, William S. 1977. *Clinical and Experimental Hypnosis in Medicine, Dentistry, and Psychology*. Philadelphia: J.B. Lippincott Co.

LeCron, Leslie M., and Bordeaux, Jean. 1947. *Hypnotism Today*. North Hollywood, CA: Wilshire Book Co.

May, Rollo. 1975. *The Courage To Create*. New York: W.W. Norton, Inc.

McKay, Matthew; Davis, Martha; and Fanning, Patrick. 1995. *Messages: The Communication Book, Second Edition*. Oakland, CA: New Harbinger Publications, Inc.

McKay, Matthew; Davis, Martha; Fanning, Patrick. 1981. *Thoughts & Feelings: The Art of Cognitive Stress Intervention*. Oakland, CA: New Harbinger Publications, Inc.

Mednick, Sarnoff A. 1964. *Learning*. Englewood Cliffs, NJ: Prentice Hall.

Murray, Edward J. 1964. *Motivation and Emotion*. Englewood Cliffs, NJ: Prentice Hall.

Papolos, Demitri, and Papolos, Janice. 1992. *Overcoming Depression*. New York: HarperCollins.

Quick, Thomas L. 1980. *The Quick Motivation Method*. New York: St. Martin's Press.

Samuels, Mike. 1975. *Seeing With the Mind's Eye*. New York: Random House and Bookworks.

Schuller, Robert H. 1967. *Move Ahead With Possibility Thinking*. Garden City, NY: Doubleday & Co.

Selye, Hans. 1956. *The Stress of Life*. New York: McGraw-Hill Book Co.

Tutko, Thomas, and Tosi, Umberto. 1967. *Sports Psyching*. Los Angeles: Westwood Publishing Co.

Wallace, Benjamin. 1979. *Applied Hypnosis: An Overview*. Chicago: Nelson-Hall.

Wolberg, Lewis R. 1972. *Hypnosis: Is It For You?* New York: Harcourt, Brace, Jovanovich.

Wolpe, Joseph, with Wolpe, David. 1981. *Our Useless Fears*. Boston: Houghton Mifflin Company.

Wyckoff, James. 1975. *Franz Mesmer: Between God and the Devil*. London: Prentice-Hall

Periodicals

Bernauer, Newton W. Ph.D. "The Use of Hypnosis in the Treatment of Cancer Patients." *American Journal of Clinical Hypnosis,* Jan. 1993.

Kangilaski, Jaan. "Dialogue: A link to psychosomatic illness." *Journal of the American Medical Association,* May 28, 1962, 2760, 2767–68, 2773.

Nelson, Mariah Burton. "Mental Workouts." *Women's Sports,* May 1984.

Rosenthal, N.E. "Diagnosis of Treatment of Seasonal Affective Disorder." *JAMA,* 270:2717–2720. 1993.

Ryan, Kathleen O. *Body Watch, Get Well Soon*: "What You Know Before Surgery Can Hasten Recovery." July 19, 1994.

Wallis, Claudia. "Unlocking Pain's Secrets." *Time,* June 11, 1984.

Some Other New Harbinger Self-Help Titles